The Baby Sleeps Tonight

Your Infant Sleeping Through the Night by 9 Weeks (Yes, Really!)

Shari Mezrah

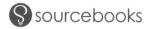
sourcebooks

Sourcebooks and the colophon are registered trademarks of Sourcebooks, Inc.

Published by Sourcebooks, Inc.
P.O. Box 4410, Naperville, Illinois 60567-4410
(630) 961-3900
Fax: (630) 961-2168
www.sourcebooks.com

Library of Congress Cataloging-in-Publication Data

Mezrah, Shari.
 The baby sleeps tonight : your infant sleeping through the night by 9 weeks (yes, really!) / Shari Mezrah.
     p. cm.
 1. Infants—Sleep. 2. Sleep-wake cycle. 3. Naps (Sleep) I. Title.
 BF720.S53M64 2010
 649'.122—dc22

                              2009046225

        Printed and bound in the United States of America.
             VP 10 9 8 7 6 5 4 3 2 1

HAYNER PUBLIC SQUARE

MAY 1 2 2010

Praise for *The Baby Sleeps Tonight*

"Shari's revolutionary new plan not only helps new moms get their babies on schedule, but also fosters a healthy attachment between mother and baby. I would highly recommend this plan to all new and expectant parents."

—CARRIE A. COHEN, CLINICAL PSYCHOTHERAPIST
AND REGISTERED PLAY THERAPIST

"Shari Mezrah's plan of creating predictability gives balance and helps to lessen postpartum-related issues, thus ensuring a happy and healthy mother and baby."

—JILL HECHTMAN, MD, FACOG

"Shari Mezrah helped our family survive the chaos of many sleepless nights with newborn twins. Enjoy the guaranteed benefits of taking control and living and feeling a balanced life with her plan."

—ANGELA GLAZER, PhD, LICENSED PSYCHOLOGIST,
FOUNDER AND CREATOR OF WWW.WHOLESOUL.COM,
AND JOEL GLAZER, OWNER, TAMPA BAY BUCCANEERS

"This program is NOT just about sleep. It's about getting your life back and taking control. Other than the fact that your child WILL sleep after this program, it allows you to be able to foreshadow and plan ahead. We can honestly say to any expectant parent or anyone out there having sleep difficulties, this is the plan for you. The program is foolproof and Shari is an angel."

— BETH EIGLARSH AND MARK EIGLARSH,
FEATURED LEGAL ANALYST ON HLN AND
FOX NEWS CHANNEL'S *THE O'REILLY FACTOR*

"As a working professional and a mom, I found The Baby Sleeps Tonight Plan to be a lifesaver! My schedule is so busy that I really don't know how I would have survived without it. Shari's positive and uplifting approach was so helpful. I truly believe that every new parent will benefit from using this plan."

— JULIE CARRUTHERS, EXECUTIVE PRODUCER
OF *ALL MY CHILDREN*

"My husband and I were at our wits' end with exhaustion! The Baby Sleeps Tonight Plan gave us a schedule to follow. By the time our daughter was nine weeks old, she was sleeping eight hours. This plan turned our lives around and we were rested and enjoying our newborn. No doubt, it helped us enjoy and make the most out of a time period where most parents are begging for more sleep!"

—Virginia Jones, PsyD

"The Baby Sleeps Tonight Plan has truly saved us. Our son adapted to the schedule immediately and sticks to it to this day. All the books regarding baby sleep and schedules were so confusing. This plan made sense and gave us so much guidance. It also gave me (a new mommy) confidence. The Baby Sleeps Tonight Plan was the answer to our 'sleep-through-the-night' prayers!"

—Ali Garrity

"As a pediatrician, over the years I have referred desperate parents to Shari for help. The results spoke for themselves: happier families that are functioning because of restful sleep. I recommend highly to all new parents!"

—Patrick C. Yee, MD

This book is dedicated to you, the parents.

Contents

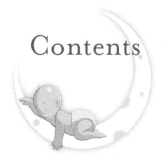

Foreword

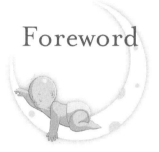

Becoming new parents was one of the most stressful times in our lives. My husband and I had just finished grueling residency training, started our medical practices, and were finally ready for a child. Then the panic hit. How would we be able to do this? How could we make sure we raised a confident, secure, and loving child? Despite the fact that I'm an OB/GYN and my husband is a general surgeon, we were terrified. We always joked that we would rather handle hemorrhaging patients than raise a child!

Then came Shari. My mother had given me a magazine article that featured Shari and how her plan could get your baby sleeping through the night by nine weeks. Our first meeting with her was when I was thirty-six-weeks pregnant, when our anxiety level was at an all-time high. Once we met her, we realized how invaluable she was on so many levels, not just sleep. Afterward, we felt incredibly empowered and ready for our challenge.

We followed her suggestions to a tee, and the plan alleviated our stress and the fear of the unknown. It gave us the knowledge of what to expect ahead of time. What's more, it worked! It was amazing.

This plan also allows for the involvement of mother and father, thereby increasing the bonding between both parents and the child. My husband wouldn't give up his 12:00 a.m. feeding for anything—it was his private moment with our daughter that he will remember forever. It made us stronger as a couple because we were truly a team. Not only does this involvement give the father a special bond with the child, but it keeps everyone sleeping longer. I was able to sleep for six hours straight from the time our daughter was born, and that made a world of difference.

As a physician, I recognize the effects that decreased sleep has on a person. When you're tired, your fuse is shorter, and you don't react in the same manner as someone who has a healthy sleep pattern. With sleep deprivation you experience changes in mood and often feel irritable. All postpartum patients are at risk for baby blues and even depression. With the change in hormone levels, we have a tendency to feel sad, tearful, lonely, and even inadequate. When you top this off with exhaustion, it really puts patients at risk. Shari Mezrah has developed a formula that alters the postpartum experiences that sometimes occur in women after birth. Her plan of creating predictability gives balance and helps to lessen postpartum-related issues, thus ensuring a happy and healthy mother and baby. By increasing the amount of sleep, you're better prepared to tolerate the physical and hormonal changes that come.

There so are many positive effects to this system. The plan is very supportive of breast-feeding, while allowing for bottle-feeding as well. There's so much talk about "nipple confusion," but as a physician, I don't believe in that. There are plenty of bottles that did not affect our daughter. Shari helped us to establish that early on. Our daughter would breast-feed from me, or my husband could give her a bottle; we had the best of both worlds. The plan also makes recommendations on how to best equip your nursery, and shares tips for teaching your baby to self-soothe.

I recommend The Baby Sleeps Tonight Plan without any reservation. I've watched my friends and the way they raise their children, and I notice a complete difference in the babies that have used this system. Looking back, I realize that with the help of this invaluable schedule, I have succeeded in my goal of creating a confident, secure, and loving child. I can see now that all of our fears while pregnant have been conquered. My husband and I truly owe our family's success to Shari's plan.

—JILL HECHTMAN, MD, FACOG, CHAIRMAN, DEPT. OF OB/GYN,
BOARD OF TRUSTEES, BRANDON REGIONAL HOSPITAL,
MEDICAL DIRECTOR/VICE PRESIDENT, TAMPA OBSTETRICS

—JASON HECHTMAN, MD, FACS, HECHTMAN SURGICAL LLC,
CHAIRMAN, DEPARTMENT OF SURGERY,
BRANDON REGIONAL HOSPITAL

Acknowledgments

In deepest gratitude I want to acknowledge my husband and best friend, Todd, for his inspiration, support, and motivation to write this book so that I can share my wisdom and innovative plan with new and expectant parents everywhere.

To my kids, Maxwell and Samantha, I appreciate both of you for your dedication to me in this endeavor, and for being the first Baby Sleeps Tonight Plan prodigies.

To my mom and dad, Ginny and Ben Puttler, who have guided me throughout my life, thank you for teaching me the love of order, time, and structure, and for always encouraging me to pursue my dreams!

I wish to thank Marci Wise for being my voice and an incredibly talented writer; my agents Sheree Bykofsky and Janet Rosen for believing in my vision of *The Baby Sleeps Tonight*; and Shana Drehs, my editor at Sourcebooks, for her guidance and expertise in the publishing of this book.

Deep appreciation to Drs. Jill Hechtman and Jason Hechtman, who have been devoted advocates of the plan from both a client and medical perspective.

I also want to acknowledge and offer special thanks to all my clients who took the time to be interviewed and share their personal stories. Thank you for your amazing support and for sharing how The Baby Sleeps Tonight Plan has changed your lives.

Most of all, I want to thank you, the parents, who have taken the first steps toward predictable happiness.

Author's Note

The content of this book has been developed by the author through years of coaching parents on sleep-related issues. However, the author is not a physician, psychological professional, or licensed counselor. The information provided in this book must not be construed by the reader as psychological, medical, or other professional advice, which can only be given by licensed professionals having an individual patient relationship. Instead, this book contains only the author's personal opinions on the topics discussed, and neither the author nor publisher of this book makes any express or implied warranty regarding the information and techniques provided, including, without limitation, the implied warranties of merchantability or fitness for a particular purpose. As with all books providing information of this kind, readers are encouraged to seek assistance from qualified professionals who can assess their particular needs.

Introduction

$\mathcal{L}$ife today is so complicated—it can be a struggle to create balance under the best of circumstances. When you add a new baby to the mix, it's no wonder many new moms become overstressed by the mind-numbing madness.

That's where *The Baby Sleeps Tonight* comes in. Packed into this pocket-sized book is a practical, progressive, and customizable approach to creating order and predictable happiness in your household—and to get baby (and the whole family!) sleeping through the night by nine weeks.

This proven formula for success includes a schedule for feedings, naps, and wake-times. You'll see that by extending the day, you can create the night. It's your first step toward becoming empowered on the wonderful journey we call parenthood.

How The Baby Sleeps Tonight Plan Was Born

I was overwhelmed after I gave birth to my son Maxwell. I'd read all the books out there and practically memorized the plans, the ideologies, the processes; yet, no one, no book, prepared me for parenthood—and the nights I spent awake. There were so many books out there and so many opinions. Whose ideas were the best? Not only was I trying to figure out how to get my son to sleep, I was also trying to calculate how to efficiently feed him in a way that adequately dealt with my milk-filled breasts, manage relationships with my family members, deal with the stress, and handle the pain in my body. And what about my spouse who was trying to work and find time to be a new parent?

I needed to take control. I needed a plan. I knew the key to the problem was getting my child's days and nights on track, so I started there and created a plan that incorporated scheduled efficient feedings, scheduled naps, and scheduled wake-times. I structured the plan so that it was easy enough for even the most sleep-deprived mom—someone like me!—to understand and implement. The result: a plan that has worked for countless families. I found myself with a confident, well-adjusted child, a child who knows he's loved, who knows when the next meal is coming, and who was sleeping eight hours straight by the ninth week of life.

And this can be your child too. Helping families is my life's passion. I'm now a sleep schedule specialist who has achieved an astonishing 100 percent success rate with families who have followed my innovative system. Over the years, I've had the privilege of sharing my successful plan with families all over the world, from single parents to families with multiples. The Baby Sleeps Tonight Plan offers a proven system for taking back control of your life, your sleep, and your happiness.

I've always been solution-oriented, and through much time and effort I've found a way around the potential pitfalls of parenthood, a strategic way to manage time so that you can enjoy the freedoms of life. The special gift that this plan provides to parents is hope and encouragement when they need it the most. We only live one lifetime, and my mission is to help you make the most out of the time that you have with your family. While my practice, BabyTIME, is located in Tampa, Florida, I regularly reach out to desperate families all over the globe through the use of my website www.sharimezrah.com and zealous referrals. The Baby Sleeps Tonight Plan is highly respected by physicians, psychologists, and, most importantly, clients, and now it's my honor to share it with you.

Unlike other baby sleep books, *The Baby Sleeps Tonight* steps back a bit from the cradle. It's my belief that baby sleep cannot be separated from the other needs in a baby's life. And I've found that the best, most effective way of meeting those needs is to keep one step ahead of them.

Predictable Happiness Defined

Predict—verb

To state, tell about, or make known in advance, especially on the basis of special knowledge.

Happiness—noun

Good fortune; pleasure; contentment; joy.

I coined the term "predictable happiness," which by definition is the ability to know what will happen next and feel good about it. The Baby Sleeps Tonight Plan is based on this concept. Why be reactionary when you can be empowered? Incorporating the plan into your family's life will lessen the degree of anticipatory anxiety you'll experience as a parent. Through a three-pronged approach of scheduled feedings, naps, and wake-times, the plan will create balance and predictable happiness in your life, while enabling everyone in the house to avoid sleep deprivation and regain their clarity and peace of mind.

THIS IS ABOUT SLEEP, ISN'T IT?

If I'm talking about all of baby's needs, is this really a book about sleep? Yes. We cannot overestimate the importance of sleep. Sleep is a necessary and vital biological function, and it's essential to a person's physical and emotional well-being. Studies have shown that without enough sleep, a person's ability to perform even simple tasks declines dramatically. For children, deep sleep coincides with the release of growth hormones, necessary for growing children.

Yet, *The Baby Sleeps Tonight* is much bigger than simply helping your child sleep through the night. What you have in your hands is a plan to help you gain control over parenting itself. Sleep is the first major hurdle to tackle, but once that's accomplished you can take the plan's positive effects even further.

The Baby Sleeps Tonight Plan will outline exact times for you, including scheduled feedings, designated naps, and sleeping through the night. You'll learn to meet your child's needs ahead of time by creating order in the household and laying the foundation for a healthy sleep environment and a happy life.

Why This Book?

I'm a mom. I've been where you are. My plan is not based on polls, philosophical ideology, or the latest craze of the moment. Instead, this is a practical guide, back to sleep and sanity, devised by a woman who has been in the trenches of motherhood.

With so many other books claiming to help you get your child sleeping through the night, how do you know which one to choose? In my opinion, it benefits everyone in your family to choose a plan that empowers you. Other sleep books encourage co-sleeping with your baby, but this plan supports independence and control by helping your child adjust to his or her own space right away. Many sleep books promote a feeding-on-demand system for the first few months of your child's life, but The Baby Sleeps Tonight Plan begins scheduling immediately, keeping you one step ahead of your baby's needs from the very beginning, and therefore putting control in your hands from day one. Other sleep books ignore the rest of a baby's life whereas this book recognizes that baby asleep is not separate from baby awake. And finally, there are sleep books out there that clock in at a whopping three hundred pages, but I designed this slim guide to be easier on a tired mom's eyes.

HOW THE BABY SLEEPS TONIGHT PLAN IS DIFFERENT

- You'll learn real solutions for getting your baby, and everyone else in the house, sleeping through the night by nine weeks.
- You can customize the plan to your family's own unique schedule.
- The plan helps to promote predictable happiness by warning against the danger of creating conditioned responses.
- Each chapter concludes with real-life success stories from parents who have used the plan.
- The plan encourages being proactive and taking back control, thereby relieving anticipatory anxiety.
- The plan offers new parents much needed peace of mind by providing helpful checklists and Motherly Advice sections that address a wide array of childcare issues.
- The chapter "Troubleshooting—Your Questions Answered" addresses areas of specific concern that new parents may face.

How to Use This Book

Time is a precious commodity when you have a new baby in the house, and The Baby Sleeps Tonight Plan is structured to give you the help you need, when you need it! While many other books for new parents are way too big and almost impossible to conceptualize when you're sleep-deprived, this one is succinct, to-the-point, and easy to use.

If you're an expectant parent, I recommend starting at the beginning of the book and reading through. However, if you've already given birth, simply go to the table at the beginning of chapter 1, find the time frame you're in right now, and skip to the appropriate page for your child's age. You'll find that the time specifics of *The Baby Sleeps Tonight* sleep schedule will become your lifeline toward creating balance, order, and sanity. Refer to them often or copy and post them in your home.

Life should be about love, laughter, and family. It doesn't need to be so chaotic that we can't enjoy the simple pleasures of a smile, a sunny afternoon, or a melody that touches our hearts. With The Baby Sleeps Tonight Plan, predictable happiness is at your fingertips! This plan will get your child sleeping through the night, and keep him sleeping through the night. It's a program that has brought peace and happiness to families all over the world.

It will do the same for you.

.... *Note* ....

The Baby Sleeps Tonight Plan is intended for full-term infants (forty weeks). If you have any concerns regarding your baby's readiness to begin a scheduling regimen, consult your pediatrician.

Chapter 1

The Expectant Parents' Empowerment Guide

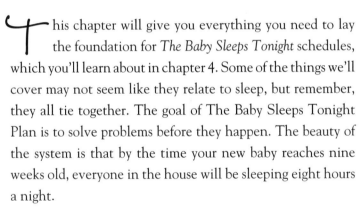

This chapter will give you everything you need to lay the foundation for *The Baby Sleeps Tonight* schedules, which you'll learn about in chapter 4. Some of the things we'll cover may not seem like they relate to sleep, but remember, they all tie together. The goal of The Baby Sleeps Tonight Plan is to solve problems before they happen. The beauty of the system is that by the time your new baby reaches nine weeks old, everyone in the house will be sleeping eight hours a night.

But there's even more sleep coming your way. As early as the tenth week, you'll reach the Ultimate Schedule in which your child will be sleeping ten to twelve hours per night. This schedule will stay with your child all the way through her toddler years.

If you're reading this book in or before your eighth month of pregnancy, congratulations! You've discovered the plan at the perfect time—you'll be able to customize the plan to your

Where to Go

If your baby is

0–3 weeks . . . . Page 61
Start at the Weeks 1 through 3 schedule

4–6 weeks . . . . Page 61
Start at the Weeks 1 through 3 schedule

6–8 weeks . . . . Page 79
Start at the Weeks 4 through 6 schedule

2–4 months. . . . . . . Page 87
Start at the Weeks 7 and 8 schedule

5–6 months. . . . . . . Page 101
Start at the Week 9 onward schedule

6–9 months. . . . . . . Page 101
Start at the Week 9 onward schedule

9–12 months. . . . . . Page 101
Start at the Week 9 onward schedule
(minus the catnap)

12–18 months . . . . Page 108
Start with the Ultimate Schedule
(minus the catnap)

18–24 months . . . . Page 108
Start with the Ultimate Schedule
(minus the morning nap and catnap)

2–3 years . . . . Page 108
Start with the Ultimate Schedule
(minus morning nap and catnap)

lifestyle and feel confident and in control before the baby is born. If you're reading this later, however, don't worry. You can jump in at any time by turning to the appropriate pages, as listed below. I'd recommend reading this chapter also, as you can save some stress by sorting out the issues we'll discuss now.

Important Areas of Discussion

Pregnancy is a time when emotions can be running high in anticipation of the new arrival. How will this baby change your life? It's important to sit down with your spouse and start planning a strategy to suit your particular lifestyle needs. You'll need to custom fit The Baby Sleeps Tonight Plan around your unique roles, responsibilities, and deadline commitments. Discussing these obligations from the beginning will go a long way toward alleviating your anxiety and get you moving on the right track from day one. Begin The Baby Sleeps Tonight Plan by discussing each of these areas with your partner:

Who will be responsible for the household chores?

It pays to be prepared! Make a list of all household duties (laundry, cleaning, shopping, lawn work, etc.) and determine who will be responsible for each. Discuss the possible scenarios that could arise and decide in advance who will handle them.

Will others be helping you during those first few weeks?

If so, be sure to include their responsibilities when mapping out your household duties list. These sorts of arrangements go much more smoothly when all involved know exactly what's expected of them. Clearly communicate the areas in which they can be of most help to you. Odds are they'll appreciate being included in this special time and be more than happy to help out.

Who will be taking care of meals in the first few weeks after you bring the baby home?

Remember, Mom will need some healing time, so planning the meals in advance can eliminate a lot of stress. There are several new businesses popping up that allow you to create two weeks' worth of meals, package them, and then keep them in your freezer until ready for use, and an array of cookbooks that show you how to cook in bulk and freeze it for later. However you choose to do it, preparing meals in advance will let you focus on what's most important: your new baby.

Who will be on call if the baby wakes in the middle of the night?

Will you take turns? Much of this will depend on whether you're breast- or bottle-feeding, or both. (We'll discuss feeding briefly on page 8, and in more detail in chapter 3, but for now just start thinking about it.) The Baby Sleeps Tonight Plan will have your baby sleeping through the night in record time, but prepare yourself now for those first few weeks when you'll be awake frequently. Just knowing that you have a formula for success will help you to navigate those early weeks with much less stress than the typical new parent.

Who will care for the older children in the household?

If this is not your first child, then ideally someone other than the mother should tend to older children for the first little while, allowing her to sleep when the baby sleeps. The first couple of weeks after delivery, it will be important for Mom to focus on healing and getting the new baby accustomed to the schedule. Usually Dad can easily take over this duty, but if you're a single mother you may need to enlist some extra help. Do you have a relative who can stay with you? If not, perhaps a good friend or hired night nurse/nanny may be the answer. Your rest is crucial in those early weeks in order to aid healing. These are the most challenging weeks for a new mother, so any help you can get is beneficial.

Grandparents

A new addition to the family generates a lot of excitement, and so many times grandparents are eager to offer their help in those first few weeks. It's important to keep the lines of communication open between you and your partner. Before you agree to allow your parents to stay with you, discuss the situation to decide if that will, in fact, be of help to you. Ask yourselves: is this the best thing for us? The first few weeks with your baby can be an overwhelming time if you're not prepared for what may be coming your way. Take the time to weigh the pros and cons and, if you decide to use their help, make sure that they're aware that you're committed to following The Baby Sleeps Tonight Plan. For this system to work, it needs to be strictly followed. Your baby's sense of well-being and the order of your household depend on it.

Naturally, most grandparents will want to do things the way they always did them in their own home, so it's important to calmly and respectfully explain why you're opting to do this program, which may be drastically different. Have a heart-to-heart conversation with grandparents to convey that you've both decided that this program is the best option for your new family. You could say, "Mom, we really appreciate your insights but we've already decided that sticking to a schedule will suit our lifestyle best, so we hope you'll support us in this." Although you may receive some resistance from them, ultimately the decision is yours and yours alone. Generally, most parents will honor your wishes once the guidelines are clearly established. Both your hormones and emotions will be running high the first few weeks after delivery so the earlier you can have this discussion with them, the better.

Once everyone's onboard with the plan, make sure to include their help in your list of duties. Their stay will be much more pleasant, and productive, if they know exactly how they can be of help to you. For example, you may want an in-law to take one of the bottle-feedings so that you can rest. If so, establish that ahead of time. It's easy to map out a guide for everyone since you'll be following the structure of The Baby Sleeps Tonight Plan. And help can mean more than just taking care of baby! There's always extra laundry that needs to be done, shopping, errands, mowing the lawn, etc. Take advantage of the help while you have it, and use that extra time to focus on getting some rest and healing.

Establishing Visiting Hours

For the last nine months you've been building anticipation in your friends, family, and co-workers as to what the little person inside you would look like. Once the baby's here they'll all want to come over and see for themselves. In order to avoid mass chaos and maintain your ability to stick with the plan, you'll need to establish specific times that you'll be accepting guests. Visiting hours should typically be broken down into two-hour blocks of time. The most opportune time to visit the baby is just after a feeding. Using the schedule as your guide, allow friends and family to visit with baby during wake-time, before he goes down for a nap. All of this can be set up ahead of time since the plan gives you a sense of predictability as to what your day will be like. For example, perhaps you'd like to schedule guests after the noon or 3:00 p.m. feedings. Having a plan allows you to find the time for the things that are important to you.

> ### MOTHERLY ADVICE:
> ### LAST TANGO IN PARIS
>
> Okay, so maybe not Paris, but you should at least take the time to visit your favorite restaurant for some special couple time before the baby is born. Even with a schedule, it will take a few weeks to get into the groove, so really treat yourselves! You're about to take your home life to a whole new level and celebration is in order. Make it a night you'll always remember.

Think about Breast-Feeding
Breast versus Bottle

Now is the time when you may want to give some thought to how you're going to feed your baby. There's no right or wrong answer here. It's true that mother's milk is full of many of the mother's antibodies that may help the baby to resist illness. For this reason, I always recommend that new mothers should educate themselves on breast-feeding and give it a try. It's important to realize, though, that breast-feeding is a work in progress. Often, we feel like we have to live up to the expectations that our mothers, and society, can sometimes place on us. If you find that you can't breast-feed you may feel like a failure. Don't allow yourself to fall into this emotional trap. The fact is that everyone's body is different, and not everyone can do it. Some women have inverted nipples that can make breast-feeding difficult; for others it may simply be that their milk doesn't come in. Not everyone's experience is the same, but I always recommend consulting with a lactation consultant before giving up. Many times they can offer helpful solutions that you may not have thought of. Whether you decide to breast- or bottle-feed is a decision that only you can make, but I usually recommend doing a combination of both. Chapter 3 will outline the benefits of each feeding approach in more detail.

Condition Your Nipples

If you plan to breast-feed, it's a good idea to start conditioning your nipples with lanolin about two weeks prior to your due date. Doing so can help you avoid pain and irritation when the baby begins to suckle. The lanolin will decrease the likelihood of dry and chafed nipples, which can make breast-feeding miserable. As always, the goal of The Baby Sleeps Tonight Plan is to cut off potential problems at the pass. Just remember to always wipe off both breasts before allowing the baby to feed. (And be careful not to overstimulate the nipples, as this can bring on labor.)

Nursery Essentials

Now's the time to put the finishing touches on the baby's room—some have been known to come early, you know! Both you and your baby will be spending plenty of time in the nursery, so take a moment to assess the readiness of the area. There are dozens of gizmos and gadgets that you can use to accessorize the room, but here I want to focus on those that are absolutely essential to baby's schedule (and baby's sleep).

A Sound Machine—It's Magic!

My favorite tool for soothing baby to sleep is a sound soother. This wonderful device can be found easily at retail stores and is an incredibly helpful tool. It's magical, and I promise that you will love it as much as your baby! The white noise function can emulate the comfort and familiarity of the environment your baby has just spent the last nine months in. That is, the sound of the room should be the sound of the womb. The sound also drowns out any other exterior noises. The key to using a sound machine effectively is to make sure that it's already on when you enter the room. If the baby hears you turn it on every time you put him down for a nap, then he'll begin to associate that sound with going to sleep (and consequently separation from you) and may learn to resist it. Ideally, you want to be in the position of control, not the baby.

The monotonous hum of the sound machine will lull your

baby into a peaceful, undisturbed sleep. Some noise is actually good for a baby. If your child always has silence, she will always need silence. Teaching your baby to embrace sound will serve as an important tool when you take her out into the busy world, where silence is impossible.

Nursing Pillow

Never underestimate the importance of things that can make your life easier. A nursing pillow—some common brand names are Boppy and My Brest Friend—is a special machine-washable pillow that can help you support the baby while nursing. It makes feeding the baby much easier while eliminating strain on the mother's back. Later it can be used as an aid for your baby's physical development. Propping your baby up on a Boppy for some "tummy time" will allow him to exercise the muscles needed to turn over and increase mobility. You can allow your baby to use the Boppy during scheduled wake-times to expend energy in preparation for a peaceful nap.

> ### MOTHERLY ADVICE: MAXI PADS
>
> Overnight diapers are great to use on your baby during the night and also for long trips—the extra absorption helps baby stay dry (and asleep) longer. If overnight diapers are not available, why not use a maxi pad placed inside of a regular diaper? My clients love using these. It's an easy way to save yourself time and trouble by using something you may already have around the house. It's great, period!

Glider Rocker

While it might not be the most fashionable piece of furniture in your home, it will certainly be among the most useful. A glider rocker is an effective tool for comforting and feeding your baby. In addition to being more comfortable and stable than a traditional rocking chair, the fluid motion of the glider's movement can help to relax both mother and baby. It's great to use in conjunction with a Boppy. These items can be in high demand by new moms so be aware that you may have to order one well in advance of your due date.

Crib/Bassinet

Ideally, I'd recommend using the crib from day one. This way, your baby is growing accustomed to her environment from the very beginning. If you're nervous about leaving your baby alone, video and audio baby monitors enable you to keep an eye on her at all times without actually being in the same room. They provide a level of security for both mom and baby while each of them gets used to the new living arrangements. However, if you've had a C-section, going back and forth to the baby's room when you've just had several layers of muscle cut may be more than you bargained for. In that case, you may have to use a bassinet. If you do, just be sure to limit its use to the first two weeks only. You can help baby transition to a crib by using familiar sounds and smells. I do not recommend co-sleeping because it's not allowing you your space, nor is it allowing your baby to become comfortable in her environment. There's plenty of time for love, cuddling, feeding, and warmth, but sleep time should be sleep time.

MOTHERLY ADVICE: RECONSIDER BABY WIPE WARMERS

Contrary to what people might tell you, baby wipe warmers are not really necessary. In my opinion, you may just be setting yourself up for a conditioned response from your baby that you don't need. Babies come to expect certain behaviors simply because that's what they're used to. Suppose you're away from home (and your baby wipe warmer) and you need to change your baby's diaper. If your baby is used to warm wipes, then odds are you'll experience some sort of distress from him when the cold wipes are applied. However, if you've always used wipes right out of the container without warming them, he will be fine because that's all he knows. Decide which hoops you want to jump through and which you don't. It's your game!

Bouncy Seat

A bouncy seat is an excellent tool not only for wake-time but for naptime as well. The vibration of the seat has a soothing effect on the baby and can be useful during a nap. I don't recommend leaving your baby in a bouncy seat for an extended period of time due to a lack of back support, but they're wonderful if used only occasionally.

Breast Pump

If you have decided to breast-feed, I recommend getting a double breast pump. This type of pump empties both of your breasts at the same time in a matter of minutes. The Baby Sleeps Tonight Plan offers you flexibility and freedom in how you choose to feed, and the breast pump helps with both of these. In the event that you're a working mom or often on the go, you can have an extra supply of milk and still stay on The Baby Sleeps Tonight Plan.

MOTHERLY ADVICE: BATHING YOUR BABY

When taking care of your baby you can get creative about using ordinary items around your home, including the kitchen sink! Giving your baby a bath in a traditional bathtub can be awkward and put a strain on your back. When your baby is small, try bathing him in the kitchen sink. It's much easier on you, the perfect size, and up at your level.

Vinyl-Free Baby Changing Pads

The first few weeks you'll find yourself constantly having to wash and rewash the crib sheets because of leaky diapers. A great time-saver that can get your baby back to sleep in minutes can be found in using vinyl-free baby changing pads. You simply place the pad underneath the baby, between the baby and the sheets, and then if the baby wets, you just replace the soiled pad with a new one. Pads are made of a soft, pliable, waterproof material that can be machine-washed and dried and can easily be found in the baby section of most stores.

Avoid changing pads that contain vinyl. Studies have shown that vinyl emits a gas that may contribute to allergies in children, as well as more severe health complications over a longer period of time

The Before-You're-Due List

Having a family broadens your horizons and gives you a whole new list of things to think about. Before the new baby arrives, here are some things that you might want to consider:

Prepare Older Children for the New Arrival

Help your older children to establish a connection with the baby by letting them feel the baby kick. Take them into the nursery to help build their anticipation. Involve them in your preparations and give them praise and credit for how helpful they are. Buy a baby doll and let the sibling practice holding, swaddling, burping, and feeding the baby. Read books with the older child about the arrival of a new baby—there are a number of great books dealing with this topic that serve to build anticipation and excitement for the new arrival. If a child is very young, you may not want him to be in the delivery room, but if you'd like your older child to be a part of the childbirth process, you could include her. Be sure to explain everything that's going on in a very clinical, medical way. By preparing older children for the new arrival, you're helping to ensure a happy homecoming where the primary emotion in the air will be excitement and not jealousy.

Hire Help, If You Can

Housecleaning services can take a huge weight off of new parents' shoulders. If you can afford one, it will be money well spent. The first few weeks will be the most important because after that time you'll have The Baby Sleeps Tonight Plan in full motion and will have more time and energy to devote to household duties.

Make a List of Your Friends

All hands on deck! With a new baby in the house, any help you can get will be appreciated. Make a list of friends who you think might be willing to help out. Think of a specific task that you would like each friend to tackle. Give them a call and ask them for their help with as much detail as possible. Most people will jump at the chance to help you. Remember, we can all get by with a little help from our friends!

MOTHERLY ADVICE:
PREPARE THE PRESENTS

Here's a suggestion of something you can do to head sibling rivalry off at the pass, and get your children's new relationship started off on the right foot. Before your delivery, buy a present for your older child from the baby! Wrap the gift and take it to the hospital with you in your overnight bag. The first time your older child is introduced to the baby, present her with the gift from her new brother or sister.

Also, in preparation for the new baby coming, Dad or the grandparents can take the sibling out to the store to buy a gift for the baby. This creates a common ground between the children, makes the older child feel included in the birthing process, and establishes that there are some very good things that come from having a new brother or sister!

Prepare Your Pets

Although the arrival of a baby is a wonderful and joyous occasion, there are other members of the household who might need some extra attention in order to better cope with the new addition—the family pets. In many instances, they were your "babies" first and may not understand what's happening. Pets with a more sensitive nature have been known to act out in destructive ways when they feel their environment has been disrupted. Taking measures to prepare your pets in advance will help to ensure your family's predictable happiness and ability to stick with the plan.

Dogs

Dogs in particular may find it confusing when a new "member of the pack" enters the scene. A dog might see the new baby as lower in the pack order and may display dominant behavior, such as growling, ears down or laid back over the head, and crouching. Initially, the animal may experience something akin to sibling rivalry when you introduce a new human baby into the household. You can minimize this feeling by working with your pet before you bring your baby home. Visit the Humane Society of the United States website at www.hsus.org for some great tips for how to prepare your pet.

Cats

Cats are less sociable than dogs and may choose to ignore the new baby altogether. One thing you can do to prepare your cat for the new arrival is to introduce baby sounds even before the baby gets there. Play a recording of a baby crying, cooing, or playing to help your cat become comfortable with an increased noise level. Over time, steadily begin to increase the volume of the recording to get your cat used to the occasional commotion that's sure to arise from having a new baby in the house.

It's also a good idea to expose your cat to musical mobiles, baby toys, and other sound-making devices ahead of time.

Get CPR-Certified

This is an essential thing for both parents to do. In fact, anyone and everyone who will be spending time with your baby, including baby-sitters and grandparents, should undergo CPR training. Not only do you owe it to your child to be able to handle any emergencies that may come your way, but having this knowledge will give you a sense of empowerment as a new parent. Classes are available at most hospitals, or you can visit the American Heart Association at www.heart.org for a list of classes near you.

MOTHERLY ADVICE:
A LETTER TO YOUR NEWBORN CHILD

The time right before your baby is born is magical. You're full of excitement and suspense imagining this person inside of you. One of the greatest gifts you can give your child is a snapshot of this moment by writing a letter. It's a time capsule in which you can express your feelings about your unborn baby and your dreams for the future. Years later, when your child is old enough to understand, present him with this memento. It will be a lasting reminder that he was wanted, anticipated, and loved!

Choosing a Pediatrician

Once your baby is born, it's good-bye OB/GYN, and hello pediatrician! Finding the right doctor for your baby is an important decision. Ask other moms their thoughts about the doctors you're considering. Also, I highly recommend interviewing potential pediatricians to find one whose philosophies are similar to your own. Following are some topics to discuss:

- What is your opinion on scheduled feedings versus feeding-on-demand?
- What's your opinion on breast- versus bottle-feeding?
- What is your approach toward medicating?
- What hospitals are you affiliated with?
- Do you accept our insurance plan?
- How hard is it to get an appointment?
- Do you have a well room and a sick room (so well children don't have to be near sick children)?
- What is your standard amount of time spent with a patient?
- How do you feel about antibiotic use?
- What is your recommended immunization schedule?

Packing for the Hospital

It's finally time to pack your bag and head off to the hospital! Being prepared for the birth is what begins the process of getting your baby sleeping through the night. Alleviating anticipatory anxiety and gaining control is the key here. In order to be comfortable and prepared, here's a list of things you will want to take along:

- **A going-home outfit.** Newborns should wear a hat to help contain their body heat. The hospital will most likely provide you with clothes for the baby (not very attractive), but if you'd like something a little more stylish you can bring your own.

- **Toiletries.** Amenities will vary by hospital, but you can be assured that it won't measure up to the comfort of home sweet home. You can make it a less sterile environment by bringing your own shampoo, soap, towels, slippers, robe, pajamas, and maternity bra. Remember, your comfort is key.

- **Pillow.** There's nothing like your own, soft pillow to make you feel at home.

- **Sound machine.** You know how much I love the sound machine! Bring it along to help the baby transition to life outside of the womb and help aid sleep.

- **Movies.** Pack your favorite flicks to help you unwind and pass the time if your labor should be long. Bring along your personal DVD player too, just in case you don't have one in the labor and delivery room.

- **Snacks.** If the thought of cafeteria food doesn't thrill you, pack a few of your own treats.

- **Lanolin.** If you're planning to breast-feed, bring lanolin to keep your nipples conditioned.

- **Reading material.** Bring books, magazines, or anything you enjoy reading to help take your mind off things.
- **Car seat.** Make sure that you are well-versed in the installation of the car seat because the hospital will not let you leave without inspecting it first.
- **Important medical papers.** Know your health history. You have to be your own advocate.
- **Call list.** Bring a list of the names and phone numbers of everyone you want your partner or designated person to tell about the arrival of your little one.
- **Camera and video camera.** Make sure the batteries are charged and you have new film and tape. You'll want to make sure to capture this special moment!
- **Cord Blood Registry kit.** If you have previously decided that you want to use this service, you'll need to bring your kit along with you now. You'll only have this one opportunity to do it, so be sure to pack the kit.
- **Aromatherapy.** The smell of essential oils can help ease the pain of labor and aid in relaxation. Clary sage is said to bring on labor contractions, and lavender is recommended for its calming properties; use your favorite scent if you like.
- **Your husband's bag.** Find out if there are accommodations for your husband to sleep at the hospital and, if so, have a bag ready for him as well.

Success Story: Scott

Scott is a financial advisor who used the plan with his two children.

I wanted to help make the transition of becoming a parent as easy as possible. My wife and I started in the third trimester, so we really had a game plan once the baby came. We started working on it right in the hospital. We knew that the sooner we got our baby on the schedule, the sooner she was going to learn to sleep through the night. Some of the added benefits were that we knew what to do when she was crying. This was like an instruction manual on what to do!

There were some very challenging times after Taylor was born. I'm not a doctor but I think every woman, whether she knows it or not, goes through some extremes in emotion after having a baby. Taylor's mom was very down at times and very up at times. Sometimes it was like I was looking at a different person. It was a roller coaster. I realized that she was going through something I couldn't understand. It was hard for all three of us, but over time we were able to work through it.

I can't say that I was always charming either. I'm sure I was short-tempered. It took a while for me to understand that there was something significant going on, and I think I was much more supportive when I realized it was something emotional with her and not something that I was doing.

The Baby Sleeps Tonight Plan helped to reduce our stress because there was more sleep. Also, by having a schedule and knowing what was coming next, we could better understand what the baby was trying to tell us. When you can solve a situation with your baby quicker, then you're less frazzled and it makes the entire daily process a heck of a lot less stressful!

My advice to new dads would be to do whatever you can to take the stress off your wife's shoulders because it's true that "a happy wife makes a happy home." By setting up a schedule you're going to reduce the stress. It will transition into a better sleep schedule far quicker than anything else. Certainly you have to be disciplined but you'll make life easier on both of you in a rapid amount of time.

The Baby Sleeps Tonight Plan has been very helpful. You actually know when your day is over and can have some time with your wife and sit on the couch or have a nice dinner. I have quite a few friends who are going through this too. I've recommended this plan, and it's been beneficial to them all!

Chapter 2

Welcome Home, Baby!

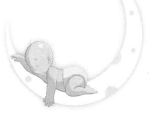

THE FIRST FEW WEEKS

They say that nothing worth having ever comes easily, and raising a family definitely falls into that category. But fear not! Most of the anxiety that affects new parents comes from being unprepared and allowing yourselves to live in a way that has you reacting to every seemingly unexpected event that comes barreling along. With The Baby Sleeps Tonight Plan we're approaching parenthood from an entirely different direction. We're making sure that you know what's coming your way, before it even gets here. We're going to make sure that you feel empowered and ready to steer your family toward predictable happiness.

Let's take a look at some of the things that new parents need to deal with in the first few weeks.

Healing Tips for After Giving Birth

It always surprises me that there's so much talk about how to give birth, but then after you've delivered, they just hand you your baby and send you on your way. There's not much discussion about taking care of you after the birth! The first step toward getting you and your family to adjust to your new life is obvious, but still many mothers underestimate its importance—you must help your body to heal. The sooner you feel better, the smoother your new schedule will become. Here are some super suggestions to help get you back on your feet in no time:

- **Frozen Tucks pads for hemorrhoids**—This can be amazingly soothing and helps to numb the pain. Dermaplast is a spray analgesic that can also help.
- **Stool softener**—Make sure you ask for a stool softener if your nurse doesn't give you one. These are especially important after a vaginal birth.
- **Hydrate, hydrate, hydrate**—Water is nature's elixir and can help a new mother in multiple ways, so drink up!
- **Granny panties**—Use the oversized, mesh panties that they give you in the hospital, or bring extra-large underwear. You'll want to be comfortable. Save your pretty panties for that special night once you've healed.

Newly Defined Household Roles

Between the constant demands of helping your baby to sleep and your need to rest and heal, the first few weeks after you get home from the hospital can be challenging. The first step toward ensuring peace and happiness for your family comes from a clear understanding of who will be responsible for certain duties in the household. Ideally, you and your husband will have already discussed this (see chapter 1) and created a plan of action, dividing up all the necessary tasks. Who will be doing the cooking? Who will clean up? If everyone knows exactly what he or she is supposed to be doing, it can alleviate anxiety and allow you to concentrate on what's most important: enjoying your new baby. If you haven't had those conversations, turn to page 3 for a list of questions to consider.

Keep Visiting Hours Reasonable

It's very important to pace yourself during those first few weeks at home. You may be riding an endorphin-high and be anxious to show off your new pride and joy, but wearing yourself out will only cause you problems in the long run. Spread out the visits and be sure to concentrate on making rest and healing your top priorities.

Using Your Time Wisely

The demands on a new mother are many. There will be times when you'll be pulled in so many directions you won't even know where to begin to place your energies. In truth, there really isn't a whole lot of extra time in the beginning. By the time you get the baby fed and back down for a nap you may only have about an hour and forty-five minutes to yourself. You need to decide how best to use that time. During the first few weeks at home, getting your rest needs to be your top priority, especially if you didn't get four to six hours of sleep the night before. Try to sleep when your baby sleeps—although it's extremely important not to allow yourself to sleep past the baby's next feeding!

Remember, on The Baby Sleeps Tonight Plan, your baby needs to be fed every three hours. Your primary goals for the first six weeks are to take care of yourself and get your baby on this three-hour schedule. If you can do that, by the end of the sixth week we can have both you and your baby sleeping from midnight to 6:00 a.m., I promise!

Okay, okay, I know what you're thinking—what about my messy house? What about all the phone messages I haven't returned? Don't worry, all those unfinished chores screaming out for attention will still be there when you wake up. Once you're feeling rested, you can begin to strategize how to use your time in the most productive manner. It's okay to have a to-do list, but be flexible about it. Know that everything isn't going to be perfect at first, but as long as you continue to work at the plan, things will eventually fall into place.

According to the National Sleep Foundation, the average adult needs seven to nine hours of sleep every night. Using The Baby Sleeps Tonight Plan will get you there as soon as physically possible, but until then, it will be up to you to make up the sleep deficit with naps.

Sleep Deprivation

What happens if your Type-A personality gets the better of you, and you start skipping naps in order to get things done? Two words: sleep deprivation. Don't underestimate the impact that sleep deprivation can have on your life. Your world can spiral out of control much more quickly than you ever thought possible. By allowing yourself to go without the necessary amount of sleep, you can inadvertently kick off a devastating chain of events. First, you may begin to rely on caffeine in order to stay awake. Unfortunately, then when you want to rest, you're not able to, and if you're breast-feeding, the caffeine definitely affects the baby's ability to sleep as well. Your emotions start to go haywire. It's very common to become irritable and lash out at others. You start to feel a general dissatisfaction with everything and don't know why. All of a sudden, you're floored by the realization that you have to take care of someone else, and you don't even know how to take care of yourself. It really is psychological turmoil.

For these reasons, it's crucially important to make your rest a higher priority than a spotless household. The National Commission on Sleep Disorders Research found that infant abuse may be more likely for sleep-deprived parents, who may feel at their wits' end and shake or hit a crying infant. Armed with this knowledge, mentally resign yourself to two months of household imperfection. By the time you and your baby get to the ninth week of the plan, you'll naturally find both energy and organization returning to your days.

The Baby Blues

If you still find yourself feeling irritable, nervous, and afraid that being a mother will never feel better than it does right now, you may be experiencing the "baby blues." After birth, your body changes rapidly. Your hormone levels drop, your milk comes in, and you may feel exhausted. The responsibilities of new motherhood can be overwhelming, and may leave you feeling weepy or moody. All of these feelings are normal during the first couple of weeks after childbirth. In fact, up to 80 percent of all new mothers experience them. The good news is that the baby blues aren't an illness and will go away on their own in about two weeks. No treatment is necessary other than reassurance, support from family and friends, rest, and time. Take special care of yourself—a massage, listening to your favorite music, or watching a funny movie can also help.

Postpartum Depression

Feelings of the baby blues that last longer than two weeks may be something more significant called postpartum depression. This state can take hold right after childbirth or several weeks or months later. The symptoms of postpartum depression are more intense and longer-lasting than the baby blues, and eventually interfere with your ability to care for your baby and handle daily tasks. According to the American Academy of Family Physicians, signs and symptoms of postpartum depression may include the following:

- Loss of appetite
- Insomnia
- Intense irritability and anger
- Overwhelming fatigue
- Loss of interest in sex
- Lack of joy in life
- Feelings of shame, guilt, or inadequacy
- Severe mood swings
- Difficulty bonding with the baby
- Withdrawal from family and friends
- Thoughts of harming yourself or the baby

Postpartum depression occurs in about 10 percent of new moms. It isn't a character flaw or weakness, but it does require prompt treatment to help you manage your symptoms and enjoy your baby. Your doctor will ask you to complete a depression-screening questionnaire and conduct blood tests to check your hormone levels. If you do find that you have postpartum depression, don't worry—you're not the first mom to get it and you won't be the last. Treatment is often a combination of counseling and medication. With the appropriate care, postpartum depression usually goes away within a few months, but it's important to continue treatment until you feel better. Stopping treatment too early may lead to a relapse.

There are many excellent resources for postpartum depression. The U.S. Department of Health and Human Services has created a website that lists telephone hotlines and support services where you can ask questions. For a list of resources visit their website at www.mchb.hrsa.gov.

In addition, The Baby Sleeps Tonight Plan can help new mothers gain control and avoid major amounts of sleep deprivation so that the symptoms of postpartum depression may be lessened.

A Father's Love

The father plays an incredibly important role in helping to get the family dynamic started off on the right foot. The key to success is to set up expectations ahead of time (sound familiar?) so that everyone knows his or her role. If Dad's working during the day, obviously that's a huge responsibility already on his plate. But whatever he can do to help will make everyone's transition much easier. Perhaps for the first few weeks Dad could bring home dinner or handle some specific chores around the house. Dads should also strive to pamper, praise, and empower their partners. Dads: while she's taking care of your new baby, it's your job to help nourish her soul.

To maximize his role in the most productive way, I recommend having Dad do one feeding a day. If he can agree to take over the midnight feeding with a bottle of breast milk or formula, it can be a huge help to Mom, allowing her to get a bigger block of sleep time and therefore greatly contributing to order in the household. Most fathers will jump at the chance to help. This feeding also allows Dad to experience closeness and bonding with the new baby. If this isn't your first baby and you have older siblings in the house, Dad will need to be on night duty for them also.

After all, Mom has just been through one of the most physically harrowing experiences of her life. She's tired, hurting, and hormonally in flux. Besides fighting a lack of sleep, her body is using an incredible amount of energy to readjust itself in order to feed the baby. Internally, there's an entire milk-making factory setting up shop. She has no choice but to go along for the ride as her body, emotions, and energy level get put through the ringer. After the first six weeks or so, a woman's body becomes accustomed to these new demands and she will rapidly begin to feel like her old self again. Knowing and anticipating this can help both parents be prepared by having realistic expectations.

If your partner has always been your knight in shining armor, you'll never know it more than at this stage of your life together. His strength and assistance are the mortar in creating a solid foundation for your new family.

Helping Siblings Adjust

Understandably, it can be hard for a young child to learn to share the affections of the most treasured people in his or her life. It's not uncommon for some jealousy to occur, but there are some things you can do to help make the transition a little easier.

Encourage Older Children to Help with Baby

You really want to make sure that the sibling feels included from the start. When the older child comes to the hospital the first time, allow him to take part in the changing of the "first diaper." Even though that may not actually be the first diaper, these sorts of rituals are important.

Create "Mommy and Me" Time

Have a designated date set up where you can have some one-on-one time with the older child while Dad watches the baby. Perhaps you could go to the park or out for ice cream. Each parent should strive to spend some alone time with the older child each day. Even as little as just ten minutes of uninterrupted time can help to prevent jealousy in an older sibling.

Your Newborn Baby and the Outside World

Even though you may be eager to introduce the newest member of your family to the world, as well as get out of the house yourself, it's important to know that very young children have an underdeveloped immune system. Newborns are generally protected by the antibodies they receive through the placenta before birth and through their mother's breast milk after birth. These antibodies will be the same ones that are circulating in the mother's system, which will include antibodies to the microorganisms in the mother's home environment and other places she frequents. As a result, babies generally have antibodies to the germs in their own homes.

However, many of the germs outside your home are foreign to both the mother and the baby, so your baby will not have antibodies to protect against these germs, and she cannot create her own antibodies against these new germs. For this reason, I recommend waiting at least two weeks before venturing out into the general population. It's in the best interest of your baby to take some precautions to make sure that she remains well. You need to be very careful about letting people touch your baby. Always make sure to carry hand sanitizer with you and use it often, because you never know what sorts of germs you may be picking up when you're out and about.

Remember, your main concentration during this time is simply setting up house. Allow yourself an adjustment period to bond with your baby, relax, and focus on your own healing.

Success Story: Liz

Liz, a former model, reflects upon life after the birth of her first baby, Max.

I got so caught up in being pregnant. I read all the books about being pregnant, but I never read any books about what happens after the baby comes. I just felt like, "Oh, we can do it. We'll have all this help from family and it'll be fine," but that was mistake number one. The first weeks were so hard, but it wasn't Max's fault; it was our fault for not being prepared.

You're living a lifestyle one day, and the next day your life changes so dramatically. That was a shock. I was sleep deprived and confused. My son was crying every two hours in the middle of the night and we would just go in there and feed him. I had no idea when he was supposed to sleep. I was reading every single book, but it was information overload. All the different opinions got so confusing. I wasn't enjoying my baby because I was too nervous and scared. I heard all kinds of conflicting advice from family and friends, and it was just too much! We had to look for help out of necessity.

Using The Baby Sleeps Tonight Plan gave me such a sense of relief. I could focus on one voice, one encouraging voice, which was so wonderful! I felt so fragile and had no confidence anymore, and having a positive voice cheering me on gave me the confidence that I needed to go on.

Lack of sleep was the hardest thing after having the baby. I see why it's used as a means of torture. You become this completely different person. It's hard to think. It's hard to make critical decisions. I would be driving and I'd keep zoning in and out and I remember thinking, "This is so dangerous for me to be behind the wheel right now."

In hindsight, I do think I had some baby blues or postpartum depression. I would hear the baby crying and my heart would start racing; I'd get out of breath and have little panic attacks and feel like "What do I do, what do I do?" And if he would go to sleep, I would feel nervous like, "When is he going to wake up? I have to tiptoe around. Oh God, oh God, oh God!" I had a lot of anxiety that I just couldn't snap myself out of.

Control, that's the basic thing. When you've got it, at least you're prepared for what may come next, whether it does or not. The minute I had the schedule I felt so much better. Having a clear plan helped more than anything. And once sleep deprivation wasn't a part of the equation, I felt like a new person.

Now my child responds well to being scheduled. I think it gives him a sense of security. He knows that after his bath his pajamas go on, and then after a sip of water he goes to bed. Now he just grabs his blanket, rolls over, and goes to sleep.

Even now, when he goes down for his nap at 9:30, he just wakes up at 11:00. I don't go wake him up—he wakes up on his own. I just marvel because I'm looking at the clock and I'll hear him start to stir and I'll just shake my head. The plan has created an internal clock within them.

Before the plan I was thinking, "Oh my God, is this going to be our life now, where every single day is going to be full of constant problem-solving?" But now we've put in the hard work and it's paying off for us. My husband and I are well-rested, we're on the same page, and we know what comes next. We feel we're better parents and happier people and that, in turn, will make Max a happier child.

Chapter 3

Feeding Frenzy

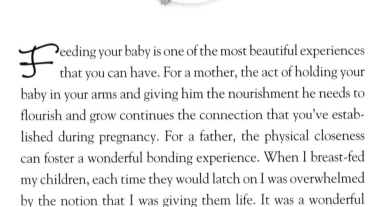

Feeding your baby is one of the most beautiful experiences that you can have. For a mother, the act of holding your baby in your arms and giving him the nourishment he needs to flourish and grow continues the connection that you've established during pregnancy. For a father, the physical closeness can foster a wonderful bonding experience. When I breast-fed my children, each time they would latch on I was overwhelmed by the notion that I was giving them life. It was a wonderful experience for me, and it can be for you too!

After months of planning for your delivery and imagining what this little person might be like, this is the moment where parenting begins; you have to teach your baby how to feed. Your baby has the instinct to feed but lacks the know-how. You are now the teacher.

It's important to note that no function in parenting is ever isolated. How your baby eats will directly affect how your baby sleeps. Naturally, when your baby is full, then she will sleep better and longer. The Baby Sleeps Tonight Plan helps you determine if your baby is being efficiently fed and therefore satisfied. It creates a "checks and balances" system to keep every area of your life running smoothly.

Breast-Feeding

Breast-feeding is a new task for both your mind and body, so there is a learning curve, but fortunately Mother Nature is happy to help out. Immediately after you give birth and begin to breast-feed, you'll notice that your milk will have a yellowish tinge, and be thick and rather sticky. This substance is called colostrum. It will take about three or four days for your breasts to produce mature milk, but in the meantime this nutrient-rich substance is the perfect first food for your baby. Colostrum is low in fat and high in carbohydrates, protein, and antibodies to help keep your baby healthy.

When your milk does come in, you may be surprised at how big and full your breasts will become. Adequate milk production is crucial to the successful breast-feeding of your baby. The Baby Sleeps Tonight Plan helps to aid milk production by scheduling the feedings at regular intervals. As we've said, the plan is all about knowing what to expect, and by feeding regularly, your body will know what to expect and respond by creating more and more of this life-giving substance! Just remember to pump your breasts on the same schedule you've got for baby's feeding, even if you're introducing a bottle of formula at the nighttime feeding. This will ensure that your milk production stays strong. You can keep those little goodie bags of milk in reserve in your refrigerator for times when you're on the go and have to use a bottle.

When breast-feeding, strive to empty both breasts at every thirty-minute feeding and don't stop to burp in between breasts. Waiting until the end to burp your baby will maintain the baby's momentum while feeding and ensure that she's taking in enough ounces.

Don't forget to apply lanolin cream to your nipples after every feeding until they're well conditioned so as to avoid pain or irritation.

MOTHERLY ADVICE: DRINK UP!

In order to help maximize your milk production, you'll need to keep yourself well hydrated by drinking plenty of water. I recommend buying yourself a water bottle and keeping it with you whenever you breast-feed. Make it your goal to drink ten to twelve ounces of water at every breast-feeding session. It's easy to put the baby's needs ahead of your own, but make no mistake about it, keeping yourself well hydrated will be of great benefit to both you and your baby.

Adding Formula

You may remember that in chapter 1 I recommended doing a combination of both breast-feeding and bottle-feeding, starting with a bottle-feeding for the last feeding of the day. I suggest using a liquid formula if available, rather than powder, because even though they have the same nutritional value, the liquid consistency is a little heavier and it will help get your baby to sleep through the night quicker.

Stress and Breast-Feeding

Believe it or not, stress can actually affect your milk supply, so it's crucially important to carve out some downtime for relaxation. Developing a practice of meditation can help. There are dozens of wonderful books on the topic, but basically meditation is simply taking the time to clear your mind, and get yourself back to a place of peace and calm emotionally. Just thirty minutes of meditation a day can do wonders for your attitude. I always say that parenthood doesn't have to be so challenging if you'll just take the steps to help yourself. Doing so allows you to feel confident and in control.

Also, children are highly intuitive and can sense your emotions. They most certainly can be influenced by your stress level and you are the barometer for the "feeling" of your family. So make every effort to maintain calm and accentuate the positive. Two of my favorite positive affirmations are

"There is nothing to fear but fear itself," and "Everything in life is manageable." If you can remember these two things, then you've already won half the battle.

MOTHERLY ADVICE: DISPOSABLE BREAST PADS

This is a great trick that can save you on laundry and embarrassment. Just insert the disposable breast pads in your bra to soak up any excess milk or lanolin. Keeping several pads in your purse or diaper bag will also ensure that you're free from any leakage accidents that may occur. (I remember being in a mall when someone else's baby started crying, and within moments my own body started responding by releasing milk. I was drenched! Disposable pads not only keep you from staining your clothing but they can also provide a breast-feeding mom a bit more confidence in public situations.)

The Breast-Feeding Diet

Once you've made the decision to breast-feed your baby, your goal is to eat high-quality, nutritionally dense food. Remember, whatever goes through you goes to the baby and therefore affects baby's sleep. Although you may love chili cheese fries, would you really want to feed that to your infant? If something irritates your stomach, you can be sure that it's going to irritate your baby's stomach as well. It's best to start testing your little one's brand-new digestive system by slowly introducing new foods one at a time. Keep a diary of what you eat and then try to draw correlations between the baby's reactions and your list. Soon you'll start to see patterns develop regarding certain foods. If your baby is more gassy and irritable than usual and is fighting bouts of diarrhea, then perhaps something you ate is the culprit. The sooner you can determine the cause, the sooner you can get on with a happy life, so it pays to take notice.

After nine months of pregnancy and packing on the pounds, I'm sure you're ready to get back to your pre-baby body. Once you've delivered your baby, your natural inclination may be to start cutting back on calories in order to meet your weight-loss goals, but I have good news for you—nature has given a reward to those who choose to breast-feed by helping you burn an additional five hundred calories per day. That's right, making milk is an exercise plan all on its own. So eat up! Combined with hearty nutrition and low-fat options, you'll automatically shed those unwanted pounds, and get your waistline back.

MOTHERLY ADVICE: BEAT THE HEAT

Night sweats can be terrible while your body is adjusting to the demands of breast-feeding. Here's a quick tip to save you time and trouble: Take an extra sheet and lay it over the spot where you sleep. If you wake up drenched with clammy sheets all around you, all you have to do is strip the top layer. Anything that buys you extra time to spend on the things that you need, like rest and relaxation, is well worth the effort. It's just one more step toward creating predictable happiness.

The No List

As adults we've come to love some things that can be very harsh on a baby's newly developed gastrointestinal system. Anything highly acidic or spicy should be introduced carefully. You should steer clear of some of these much-loved troublemakers:

- Caffeine (If you just have to have a cup of coffee, then I recommend only one cup in the morning. Coffee is a stimulant, and it will stimulate your baby.)
- Broccoli
- Garlic
- Curry
- Onions
- Leafy vegetables

- Cabbage
- Carbonated beverages
- Orange juice
- Cranberries
- Chocolate
- Sugar
- Peanuts
- Red wine
- Beer

MOTHERLY ADVICE: MEDICATION

If you have to take medication, even something over-the-counter, remember that everything that goes through you goes to the baby. It's always a good idea to make sure that any medications are approved by your doctor or pharmacist ahead of time.

The Yes List

Before you get discouraged about all the things you can't eat, know that there are plenty of well-loved favorites that you can scarf down guilt-free now that you're breast-feeding. Beefing up on protein and carbohydrates is a great idea. Protein serves as energy, and carbohydrates are associated with many of the comfort foods that we've come to love. Eating healthily will not only help you develop your milk supply but will also ensure that your baby is getting a top-quality food source.

- Protein (chicken, beef, and fish) Hard-boiled eggs are a fabulous source of protein. If you're concerned about the yolk, make an egg salad sandwich out of egg whites. It tastes terrific and is high in protein and low in fat.
- Mashed potatoes
- Bran muffins
- Rice
- Sweet potatoes
- Puddings
- Jell-O
- Macaroni and cheese
- Dairy
- Eggs
- Water
- Mother's Milk tea
- White wine (There are many negatives associated with alcohol consumption. I do believe that relaxation is important for a new mother, however. Just remember, everything in moderation! If you choose to have a glass of white wine after dinner—red wine is too full of sulfites and high acid levels—I would suggest that you be prepared to "pump and dump" at the next feeding. Feed your baby either formula or breast milk that has been previously stored. Remember, what goes through you goes to the baby, so why take a chance?)

MOTHERLY ADVICE:
MOTHER'S MILK TEA

If you feel that your milk supply starts to dwindle, you may want to consider Mother's Milk Tea. Many people swear by this tea, which is an herbal remedy generally consisting of fenugreek, fennel, nettle, and/or blessed thistle. If you do decide to turn to herbal products, I would strongly advise speaking with your doctor and doing some of your own research beforehand. It's important to note that even though they are readily available at health food stores, herbal remedies are not regulated by the FDA.

Bottle-Feeding

Human beings are naturally adaptable. If you introduce a bottle to your baby early on, she is much more likely to accept both breast and bottle without objection. If you haven't done both from the beginning, then you might have to allow your baby a little adjustment time. Every baby latches on differently and the nipple on a bottle will feel different to the baby from your own nipple. When introducing a bottle to an older baby, start with the feedings that happen earlier in the day. The baby will be hungrier and therefore more determined to make it work. As with everything, practice makes perfect, so keep trying.

Another good thing about using a bottle is that it gives

you a better visual of how much your baby is taking in. If you're breast-feeding and it's becoming a constant challenge to stretch out the time before the next feeding, then perhaps your milk is running out later in the day. Try hydrating yourself by drinking more water and supplement the baby's feedings with formula or stored breast milk. Examine all the variables to determine what may be the cause.

Formula for Success

There are several very good formulas on the market today. I would recommend using a lipid-enhanced formula, or LIPIL. These formulas are the closest in composition to breast milk and have been supplemented by two fatty acids, DHA and ARA, which are thought to promote visual and mental development in infants. Some popular brands are Enfamil LIPIL, Similac Advance, and Gerber Good Start, and there are soy formulas available as well. However, just as the breast-feeding mom observes her baby for reactions, the bottle-feeding mom must do the same. Everything is new to your baby's immature digestive system. It's not uncommon to sample a few brands of formula before finding one that works for your particular child. This is a trial-and-error process. If your baby is experiencing gastrointestinal distress, skin eruptions or rashes, and spitting up excessively, this could be a reaction to the formula you're using. Alert your pediatrician to the specific symptoms your baby is exhibiting and he or she will recommend an alternative formula that will better serve your baby's needs. Keep in mind, though, that constantly changing formula doesn't allow the baby to get used to one thing, so once you find a suitable brand, stick with it.

When choosing a bottle for your baby, your primary concern should be finding one that eliminates extra air consumption. I've found the Playtex VentAire Advanced bottle system to work nicely. These reusable bottles have patented technology that vents air at the back of the bottle as opposed to the nipple. There are several other bottle types available, including "drop-in" liners that don't require regular sterilization. You can do your own testing to find out what works best for your baby.

When choosing a bottle for your baby, look for one that's BPA-free. Early studies have shown that the chemical bisphenol-A, found in some plastics, could cause behavioral changes in babies or contribute to early onset of puberty in girls. The exact effects of BPA on humans aren't completely clear at this time, but it never hurts to be on the safe side. Make sure there's a BPA-free logo on the packaging before buying a bottle for your baby.

How Much Should I Feed My Baby?

There's no set and definitive answer to this question, since each baby will eat according to his or her growth rate.

Some days your baby will eat more, other days, less. People have different appetites, and babies are no different. The important thing is to ensure that your baby is receiving adequate nourishment.

Here's a rough rule of thumb for approximating how much you should be feeding your baby in a given day: If your baby isn't eating any solid foods yet, then you should offer two and a half ounces of formula per pound of body weight each day. For example, if your baby weighs twelve pounds, then you should be feeding your baby approximately thirty ounces over a twenty-four-hour period.

Your Guardian Angel: A Mother's Intuition

Although there is no scientific gauge to calculate this phenomenon, a mother's intuition is undoubtedly real. You'll have a sense of whether your baby is satisfied after eating. Don't ignore this feeling. It's nature's way of helping you along. When in doubt, seek the advice of your doctor, but never ignore your hunches when it comes to your baby.

MOTHERLY ADVICE: SPORTS BRAS

Nursing jogging bras are wonderful for breast-feeding. They unhook from the top down (making it easier to breast-feed), they offer extra support, and they're comfortable to sleep in. Just be sure to get one a size larger than you'd usually wear to accommodate your growing bustline.

Fighting Fussiness and Gas

When it comes to your baby, gas is the enemy! Even with the perfect diet and a well-tolerated formula, babies will need to be burped correctly after each feeding. If not, it will affect baby's sleep. Here are some tips that may help:

- To reduce air consumption, avoid feeding your baby in a horizontal position. It's always better to prop your baby up at an angle instead.
- Wait until your baby is completely through eating before burping. In other words, allow him to finish the entire bottle, or if breast-feeding, empty both breasts before attempting to burp him.
- When ready to burp your baby, hold him vertically on your shoulder. Make sure his diaphragm is pressed against your breastbone, creating a hard surface.

- Rhythmically pat and rub your baby's back with a firm hand, to work up any gas bubbles.

Fussiness in babies is nothing new. Over the years, the labels for stomach upset have changed and it seems that certain "trends" take center stage and then die out. For a while, everyone was talking about "colic," and today the catch phrase seems to be "acid reflux." Although having a label for your baby's distress can be comforting to a new parent, I suggest assessing all the variables to find out why the baby is crying. If you can help it, don't get into the mind-set of treating the symptoms and ignoring the cause.

For example, I recently had a client whose baby had been taking medication for acid reflux for three months. By examining all the variables of the baby's diet, we concluded that the baby's formula was actually causing the problem. After switching to a more tolerable formula, the baby was able to discontinue use of the medication.

Of course, you need to take your doctor's advice into consideration, but use your own mother's intuition, as well. On the following page are some "labels" you may hear regarding your baby and what they mean.

Colic

Colic is defined as uncontrollable crying in an otherwise healthy baby. Doctors look for a "three" pattern when diagnosing colic: more than three hours a day, at least three days a week, for at least three weeks in a row. Infantile colic usually begins at about two to three weeks of age, reaches its peak at two months, and is gone by four months of age.

Gastroesophageal Reflux Disease (GERD)

This occurs when babies consistently spit up or vomit. More than half of all babies experience acid reflux in the first three months of life. Most stop spitting up between the ages of twelve and eighteen months. In a small number of babies, certain symptoms may necessitate medication. Following are some worrisome signs to look for:

- Poor growth due to the inability to hold down enough food
- Refusal to eat due to pain
- Blood loss from acid burning in the esophagus
- Breathing problems

Contact your pediatrician if you feel your baby may be experiencing these symptoms. He or she may suggest medication that will help protect your baby's esophagus from damage due to reflux (though it is unlikely to completely cure the spitting up). If prescribed, be sure to clarify with your pediatrician how long your baby will be expected to take the medication.

MOTHERLY ADVICE: BICYCLE AWAY THAT GAS!

If your baby seems overly irritable and not sleeping, perhaps excess gas is the problem. Lay your baby on his or her back and carefully move her legs in a circular motion as if she were riding a bicycle. You may also gently push her legs up to her tummy and back down. This is a great exercise for your baby that you can do at any time during the day, but it's wonderful in helping her release excess gas as well.

Success Story: Julie B.

Julie is a working mother of two.

I found acclimating to life as a new parent a big adjustment. It was scary and very overwhelming. I was probably getting four hours of sleep a night, but not consecutively. Sleep is so important because it supplies you with energy to take care of everybody. When you don't get it you feel out of whack and depressed.

I'd read so many studies about how nutritious breast-feeding is, and I really wanted all that benefit for my children, but I just couldn't do it. People put so much pressure on you with breast-feeding, even right in the hospital. They make you feel like if you can't master it then you're going to be the worst mom. When I wasn't successful at it, I just felt terrible. I felt like a failure. That, along with the fact that I couldn't sleep, and knowing that I had to go back to work right away, was overwhelming. I was so guilt-ridden about not being able to do it, but I can honestly say that both of my children are strong, healthy, and secure, so I don't think it hurt them in any way. I just wish there wasn't so much societal pressure to breast-feed, because I think that just puts an undue burden on mothers.

I met Shari at a Christmas party and we were talking. I didn't even know what she did, but I pretty much broke down from a lack of sleep. I explained that I had a new baby at home. She said "Oh my goodness, you've got to come speak with me. I've helped a lot of people and I can help you too!" My husband and I met with her and told her that our five-week-old wasn't sleeping at all. We were willing to try anything! In three weeks time, our baby was sleeping eight hours a night! I brag about it all the time. All my friends are jealous of our luxurious sleeping schedule. They think we're the luckiest people in the world. I love it!

My advice would be to start the plan as early as you can. The schedule provides you with the knowledge that you will need to get through it. It will teach your child to self-soothe and sleep according to your life's demands. There's so much fear of the unknown when you have a baby, and it's perpetuated by there being too much information out there. You just have to stick with one thing.

Our second child is even better because we started the plan

right in the hospital. He sleeps like an angel. My twin sister had a baby four months after my son was born. She doesn't use a schedule, and now her daughter is almost a year old and still not sleeping through the night!

The Baby Sleeps Tonight Plan provides such confidence because it's a tried and true system. It's worked with two completely different children impeccably. Using the plan as a tool is essential when dealing with all the other stressors of parenthood. I can't say enough about it. I probably would have been in the sanitarium if I hadn't met Shari and used this plan!

Chapter 4

Weeks One through Three

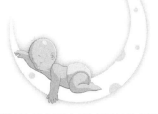

BEGINNING THE BABY SLEEPS TONIGHT PLAN

*W*elcome, baby!

Now that you've learned some of the basics about bringing baby home and feeding, we can get started on the schedule that will ultimately lead to your baby sleeping through the night by nine weeks of age. The first three weeks with your new baby are very important because that's when your family begins to find its rhythm. At this stage of the game we're not worried about getting your baby's days and nights on track, we're just getting into the rhythm of our feedings.

The Feeding Schedule

In the beginning, your feeding schedule is every three hours, just like clockwork, beginning at 6:00 a.m. The scheduled times in this book are structured to accommodate an eventual—by the ninth week—wake-time of 7:00 a.m., but you can customize the schedule to meet your specific needs. For example, if you'd like your baby to have an eventual wake-time of 8:00 a.m., then you would simply add one hour to each of the designated times outlined as follows. The key to reaching these goals is to keep the time in between feedings consistent with your specific stage of the plan.

Weeks 1 through 3 Feeding Times (Every 3 Hours!)

6:00 a.m.	6:00 p.m.
9:00 a.m.	9:00 p.m.
12:00 noon	12:00 midnight
3:00 p.m.	3:00 a.m.

In the Hospital

Ideally, you'll want to get the baby on this three-hour feeding schedule as soon as possible, even in the hospital if you can. Your specific medical situation will dictate much of what you can do those first few days, but it's important to know that even in the hospital you still have choices. Discuss your wishes with your doctor and nurses and then come as close to the schedule as you can. The hospital staff is usually more than happy to help accommodate your wishes.

Keep in mind that your hospital stay may be the only chance you'll have to rest for a while, so take advantage of it. If you've had a C-section or a very hard labor and delivery and are exhausted, ask the nurses if they can take the baby to the nursery so that you can rest. Find out when the nurses are scheduled to check your vital signs and see if you can coordinate the baby's feedings with that. With clear communication, everybody's happy—you get to rest and the baby gets fed on time.

> ### MOTHERLY ADVICE:
> ### THE NURSES ARE YOUR FRIENDS
>
> The nurses on the floor will be your advocates for those first couple of days. Granted they're very busy taking care of several patients at once, but if you let them know your desires they'll be as helpful as they can. Their support toward you and your new baby is crucial to the plan, so show them your appreciation. Plan ahead of time to have your husband bring them a huge batch of cookies as a thank you for their time and consideration. Everyone likes to be treated nicely and nurses are no different!

Goal #1
Aim for a thirty-minute feeding.

Hopefully you were able to begin *The Baby Sleeps Tonight* feeding schedule before you even left the hospital, but if not, now is the time. Your goal is to feed your baby for thirty minutes. That amount of time should be sufficient to drain each breast (fifteen minutes on each) or take a bottle. At first, this might seem like a lofty goal since your baby is just learning how to feed, but remember this is a work in progress. With each feeding, strive to feed for at least thirty minutes but no longer than one hour. Your biggest challenge at this stage of development will be keeping your baby awake.

Wake Up, Baby!

The key to keeping the baby awake is to make her feel a little bit uncomfortable by using what's known as a stimulation technique. There are several ways that you can nudge your little one out of the sleepy state:

- Undress the baby.
- Change his diaper.
- Tickle her feet.
- Blow kisses in his face.
- Put cool droplets of water on her forehead.
- Take him outside or into a brightly lighted room.
- Keep her vertical.
- Give him a bath.
- Lay her on her tummy for some tummy time.

Goal #2
Gradually increase your baby's wake-time after the feedings.

Your second goal is to keep your baby awake for fifteen minutes after the feedings (except for the feedings at midnight and

3:00 a.m.) by the end of week three. We're going to build up to fifteen minutes in small increments of time. During the first couple of weeks, try to keep your baby up for just five to ten minutes after a feeding, then put him down for a nap. He'll naturally want to sleep because that's all he knows. At this stage, infants have no concept of day and night. You wouldn't believe how many parents are unprepared for this. So many of my clients come to me and say they just thought their baby would go to sleep at 8:00 p.m. and sleep through the night. Unfortunately it's not quite that easy.

Building up to fifteen minutes of wake-time should be done gradually, adding a little more time each week. You can follow this example:

- **Week #1:** 30 minutes of feeding + 5 minutes additional wake-time = 35 minutes total wake-time, then put down for a nap.
- **Week #2:** 30 minutes of feeding + 10 minutes additional wake-time = 40 minutes total wake-time, then put down for a nap.
- **Week #3:** 30 minutes of feeding + 15 minutes additional wake-time = 45 minutes total wake-time, then put down for a nap.

In order to get baby's days and nights on track, we're working toward a progression of feeding time, wake-time, and then naptime. Here's the secret to our success and the theme of

The Baby Sleeps Tonight Plan: by extending the day, we can create the night. You can do it!

Preparing Baby for the Nap

Before putting your little one down for a nap, you'll want to make sure your baby is properly prepared. You should start prepping for the nap at least fifteen minutes beforehand, by allowing some wind-down time. During this period, limit any kind of stimulating activity. Make sure the baby's diaper has been changed and start the magic of the sound machine in the baby's room before entering. If you have a glider rocker, its rhythmic motion can be very comforting for a baby. Help baby get in the sleepy zone by holding him, rocking him, and using baby massage to relieve any gas pains. When it's time for the nap, asleep or not, put him down in the crib and walk out of the room. If he starts to cry, wait ten minutes before returning.

Tips for the Early Weeks

"Do I really need this program? Our baby is such a great sleeper!"

I hear these famous last words from almost all new parents when they first come home from the hospital. Babies do sleep a lot in the beginning. Parents begin to think that it's going to last forever, but then comes the big surprise: after about two weeks, your baby wakes up! All of a sudden, he sleeps all day and is up all night. That's why it's so important to start The Baby Sleeps Tonight Plan from day one.

> ### MOTHERLY ADVICE:
> ### *BABY MOZART*
>
> To help stimulate your baby during wake-time, try using the *Baby Mozart* series. Created by mother and teacher Julie Aigner-Clark, *Baby Mozart* is an introduction to Mozart's beautiful music. The images of brightly colored toys and objects aid in the audio presentation of child-friendly arrangements and sound effects. These DVDs can be used with children up to three years of age. Although the eyesight of very small babies isn't fully developed yet, they can still see the movement and hear the beautiful melodies. *Baby Mozart* DVDs are available on www.amazon.com or at your local bookstore.

Getting Mom to Bed

As we said earlier, the key to successfully implementing the plan is to make sure that all members in the household know exactly what's expected of them. Fathers can understandably feel left out amid the confusion of a changing household, but dear old dad is perfectly poised to swoop in and save the day by doing just one thing. If Dad can just commit to taking on the midnight feeding by using a bottle of breast milk or formula, then we can get Mom sleeping five or more hours right off the bat.

Even if you're breast-feeding, I always recommend supplementing with one bottle of formula or breast milk daily (ideally, the last feeding of the day, the midnight feeding). There are several reasons for this. Not only does it allow Dad to take an active part in the child care, as we've just discussed, but it also gives you some flexibility, helps you accumulate a supply of pumped breast milk, and gives you some time to rest.

It works like this: as soon as Mom has breast- or bottle-fed the baby at 9:00 p.m., she gets ready for bed. We want her to get to sleep before 10:00 because she's going to have to be up at 3:00 a.m. for the next feeding. Right before bed, Mom needs to do a last pump of her breasts so that she can be comfortable until 3:00 a.m. It's crucial that she sets her alarm and doesn't miss this 3:00 a.m. feeding for the first three weeks. This is an important step in getting your baby to adapt to the cycle we're creating. I've had clients for which the father can't do the midnight feeding and would prefer to do the 9:00 p.m. feeding instead. That's fine, but in doing so, Mom needs to go to bed earlier because she's going to be up both at midnight and 3:00 a.m.

MOTHERLY ADVICE:
TWINS ARE DOUBLE THE PLEASURE

If you've been given the better of two worlds and have twins to take care of, you can still use The Baby Sleeps Tonight Plan. You have a couple of choices. If you have additional help in your home, you can keep both babies on the same time schedule. If you're by yourself, simply stagger each baby's schedule by thirty minutes in order to avoid the chaos of trying to feed two babies at once.

The Crying Controversy

In 1986, Richard Ferber, the author of *Solve Your Child's Sleep Problems*, popularized the technique "Ferberizing" or allowing your baby to "cry it out." Although this method is controversial because it can be seen as rather heartless by some, there is no hard evidence that allowing your baby to cry it out causes long-term problems. While I like Ferber's methodology and do believe it's in the child's best interest to learn to self-comfort, I've developed a "Crying Checklist" to make sure that all the baby's immediate needs have been met, prior to putting him down. My mind-set, as it is with everything in The Baby Sleeps Tonight Plan, is to try to keep one step ahead of the baby. If you can do that, and be sure that your baby's needs have already been met, then you can proceed with The Baby Sleeps Tonight Plan with much greater peace of mind. In order to make sure your baby is indeed comfortable, do a mental run-through of the Crying Checklist.

The Crying Checklist

- Was the baby's diaper changed recently?
- Did the baby feed efficiently at the last feeding?
- Could the baby be too cold or too warm? (I recommend 75 degrees.)
- Was the baby burped?
- In older babies, is the baby teething?
- In newborns, is the baby swaddled?
- Is the baby sick?

If all of these criteria have been met and your baby is still crying, it's reasonable to conclude that the baby is crying because that's the only way she knows how to communicate. In time, you'll become so familiar with your baby's cries that you'll be able to distinguish between them just by their pitch and sound quality. A shrieking cry is from pain such as gas, for example. A different cry may be from hunger.

If you must go into your crying baby's room at a time other than feeding time, I warn against taking him out of the crib. That can start an undesirable cycle of conditioning: when baby cries, baby gets picked up and baby stops crying. It doesn't take long for the baby to realize that in that scenario, he wins. If he cries long enough and hard enough, Mommy will come. We're trying to eliminate that kind of conditioning and teach the baby how to self-soothe himself back to sleep.

> ## MOTHERLY ADVICE:
> ## THE WARMTH OF THE WOMB
>
> Swaddling is a technique that is a must for all newborns. To swaddle your baby, carefully lay your baby down on her back on a blanket, fold the blanket up over her feet, snugly around one side, and then around the other side, tucking the corners in, in order to re-create the warmth of the womb. This is important during the first couple of months as your baby is becoming accustomed to her new environment. It will help your baby to feel more secure and therefore sleep more soundly. This is wonderful until about the age of eight weeks, when she will be begin to break out of the swaddle due to increased mobility.

Techniques for Soothing

The key to helping babies learn to self-soothe is to satisfy their five senses, while being as minimally invasive as possible. The idea is to avoid having to pick the baby up. Try using the following techniques to help give your baby a sense of security.

Satisfy the Senses
Touch

Although I recommend not picking your baby up from the crib, you can provide comfort by reaching in and gently rubbing, patting, or massaging the baby until she falls asleep. Also, make sure that the baby is swaddled if under eight weeks old.

Sound

Your magic sound machine should already be going. White noise is proven to help children fall asleep and stay asleep, and also the rhythmic beat or gentle lull of music can help. Keep some of your favorite songs and lullabies on CD in the nursery. You can also whisper positive verbal affirmations to your baby to help him wind down. Repetitive words are often helpful. For example, "You're okay, Sam," or "Mommy loves Maxwell."

Smell

For babies who are craving connection with their mother, it may be helpful to place an item carrying her scent, such as a small article of clothing, tied to the rail of the crib. Be careful to make sure that the item is securely fastened and doesn't have any parts that baby could become entangled in.

Sight

Make sure the lighting in the room is dim and properly conducive to a sleeping environment. In addition, having a ceiling fan over the crib, running on the lowest setting, can provide a visual focal point for your baby.

Taste

Non-nutritive sucking can calm a baby's nerves. A pacifier is fine as long as it's used just occasionally so that your baby doesn't become dependent upon it. The more a child can learn to pacify herself, the better it is for everyone in the long run.

The Shirley Hold

When attempting to soothe and relax your little person, nothing works better than the "Shirley Hold." I named this technique after my nanny Shirley, who first showed me how to lull my baby into a calm and peaceful state. Here's how you do it: Lay your baby along your forearm and place the back of the baby's head into the palm of your hand. Use your other arm as additional support so that the baby is securely balanced. Gently begin to sway your arms, and the baby, in a side-to-side and back-and-forth motion. The effortless glide of the motion will feel amazingly soothing to your newborn and have a calming effect.

Recap

To recap, for the first three weeks you want to strive toward scheduled feedings of no more than thirty minutes, and you want to keep your baby awake for fifteen minutes after the feedings by the end of the third week (except for the bedtime feedings), for a total of forty-five minutes of wake-time. Those are your goals.

At midnight and 3:00 a.m. there's no wake-time; we're creating that night.

Goals: By the End of Week 3

Begin Feeding Time	End Feeding Time	Begin Naptime
6:00 a.m.	6:30 a.m.	6:45 a.m.
9:00 a.m.	9:30 a.m.	9:45 a.m.
12:00 p.m.	12:30 p.m.	12:45 p.m.
3:00 p.m.	3:30 p.m.	3:45 p.m.
6:00 p.m.	6:30 p.m.	6:45 p.m.
9:00 p.m.	9:30 p.m.	9:45 p.m.
12:00 a.m.	12:30 a.m.	
3:00 a.m.	3:30 a.m.	

Note

If your baby deviates from the schedule, don't worry. Resume the original schedule when you can, and stick to it as closely as possible, and you'll be right back on track in no time.

MOTHERLY ADVICE:
SCHEDULING YOUR DOCTOR'S VISITS

If you want to ensure a timely doctor's appointment (and thus keep on your schedule), try to get either the first appointment of the day or the first appointment after lunch. Doctor's offices tend to be less busy at these times and your wait period will be shortened considerably.

Success Story: Julie S.

At the end of her rope, Julie turned to The Baby Sleeps Tonight Plan in desperation when her first child was nine months old.

My advice to new moms would be to get your kids on a schedule as quickly as possible. When you're sleep-deprived and feeling helpless and hopeless, you need someone to tell you what to do.

I don't think women admit to each other that parenthood is hard. If you see a woman with a new baby and you ask how everything is, she always says, "Oh, it couldn't be better, it's the best!" And I thought, "This isn't the best, it's hard!" I think there's this feeling that you're betraying your baby if you say that it's not the best.

So now I try to be honest about it. When my friends tell me they're pregnant I say, "Oh, my condolences!" Then we laugh about it and I immediately recommend starting a schedule.

Even at nine months, my son was up three times a night nursing, and it was horrible! At that time we lived in a two-bedroom condo and we were so paranoid about upsetting the neighbors that as soon as he would cry we would just run and grab him. I was so sleep-deprived that I was constantly crabby and crying very easily. When I get tired, I start to withdraw and I don't really want to deal with other people. It was starting to affect my marriage.

We live in Chicago, but just happened to be in Tampa where Shari's office is located, and things had gotten so bad that we decided to meet with her. I always said my son was just a bad sleeper, that was my excuse, but Shari said there's no such thing. She said that children just crave a schedule. At that point we felt like we had nothing to lose by giving it a try. She said, "You have to start tonight!" Being away from home, we were reluctant, but she insisted, so we did and by the time we got home, three days later, he was already on a schedule!

That first night we had to keep him up late, until 11:00 p.m. in the hotel room. My husband and I were both exhausted, but then we thought, "Okay, this is three nights of our whole lives, and after that he'll sleep." The first night he actually slept from 11:00 p.m. to 6:00 a.m., which was like a miracle! Then we kept moving bedtime back until he was sleeping from 8:30 p.m. to 6:30 a.m. And it wasn't like we even had to let him cry it out, like you hear about. We were just keeping the baby up so that he was good and tired. He must have been craving a schedule because it happened so quickly. It was probably even better for him than it was for us!

I think this plan takes the best of all the advice that's available and puts it into practical steps so you can have your life back. It's not just about sleep to me because it incorporates diet and other aspects of how to live your life.

I was nursing and she even gave me instructions about things that I was eating that might be affecting the baby. Sometimes I would eat a bowl of broccoli for dinner and she told me that would upset his little stomach. That was something that nobody had ever mentioned before.

With my second child I started to talk to Shari before he was even born. Normally you would just say I'll sleep when the baby sleeps, but with a second baby that's not going to work, because you've got another one who's downstairs taking apart the TV or something.

With our second baby we were in control of the situation, we knew what to do, and we managed it. From the beginning we had the feeling of control instead of constantly reacting. I never had that feeling of hopelessness the second time around because I was using the plan right from the start. We know what we can do and when we can do it. It's allowed us to have a life!

Chapter 5

Weeks Four through Six

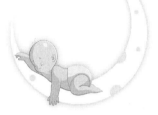

CREATING THE NIGHT

*N*ow that you've successfully tackled the first month with your new baby, your life is starting to fall into a balanced routine. Your body is still healing but you are beginning to see the benefits of The Baby Sleeps Tonight Plan. By the end of week six, your baby will be ready to sleep for six hours straight!

Weeks 4 through 6 Feeding Times
(Every 3 Hours—Drop the 3:00 a.m. Feeding)

6:00 a.m.	6:00 p.m.
9:00 a.m.	9:00 p.m.
12:00 noon	12:00 midnight
3:00 p.m.	

Goal #1

Get baby to sleep from midnight to 6:00 a.m.

Now that we're at week four, the first change in our schedule occurs: the elimination of the 3:00 a.m. feeding. Your goal in weeks four, five, and six is to get your baby sleeping from midnight to 6:00 a.m. If your baby should wake at 3:00 a.m., delay going into his room for fifteen minutes. This may seem like a long time but there's a good possibility that your baby will go back to sleep on his own. That is our objective. As a parent it may be very challenging to allow your baby to cry at first, but this stage is only temporary. If we do our job right, your baby will learn to soothe himself. When you do enter the room, give him a full feeding and then put him right back to bed. Over the next week, when your baby wakes during the night, progressively delay your response time by another fifteen minutes.

By extending the night in fifteen-minute increments, by week five your baby will typically be sleeping until about 4:30 a.m. Since you are now so close to the regular 6:00 a.m. feeding, decrease the amount of formula or breast milk at the 4:30 a.m. feeding to just enough to bridge the gap to the 6:00 a.m. feeding. An ounce or two or breast-feeding for five minutes should be just enough to get baby to go back to sleep.

Watch out—this is the danger zone! It's easy to get stuck here if you're not careful. Your baby could easily become accustomed to this short feeding, so we want to discourage that by getting past this benchmark as quickly as possible. Continue to gradually extend your response time by fifteen minutes nightly in order to condition your baby to go to sleep on his own. You can assist by using rhythmic patting and shushing techniques.

More Soothing Techniques

One of the most important discoveries you can make when attempting to soothe a crying baby is that it's all about the beat. Babies aren't used to being still. Their whole uterine existence was a moving experience. Simulating that environment can calm a fussy baby. They love a rhythm, and a gentle bouncing motion can be a huge comfort to a little one who is feeling agitated. Making a repeated shushing noise, such as shh…shh…shh…shh…shh, simulates the whooshing noise caused by the blood flowing through the mother's arteries. Rap music is also good, as the low bass sound is similar to what they heard in the womb as you were walking.

As we've already discussed, there are many benefits to teaching your baby to fall asleep with sound. Let's face it, we live in a bustling and busy world and if the only way we can fall sleep is to be surrounded by complete quiet then we might not be sleeping very much! Babies are already accustomed to hearing repetitive sound from those months in their mother's womb. Allowing your baby to use sound to soothe herself also helps your baby to transition socially. In tracking my clients who've done so, they can go out to a busy restaurant and enjoy a nice dinner while baby sleeps peacefully in the carrier beside them, undisturbed by the noise. Noise is good for a baby!

Goal #2
Gradually increase your baby's wake-time after the feedings.

Your second goal is to keep your baby awake for thirty minutes after the feedings (except for the midnight feeding) by the end of week six. Just as we did for the first three weeks, we're going to build up by five minutes each week:

- **Week #4:** 30 minutes of feeding + 20 minutes additional wake-time = 50 minutes total wake-time, then put down for a nap.
- **Week #5:** 30 minutes of feeding + 25 minutes additional wake-time = 55 minutes total wake-time, then put down for a nap.
- **Week #6:** 30 minutes of feeding + 30 minutes additional wake-time = 60 minutes total wake-time, then put down for a nap.

Recap

Before we can move on to the next stage, and our eventual wake-time of 7:00 a.m. (by nine weeks), we need to master midnight to 6:00 a.m. first. That's our primary goal in weeks four, five, and six. By delaying your response time, little by little, your baby will begin to adjust to the extended night. And if your baby has consumed four ounces of formula or had a full breast-feeding at bedtime (midnight), then there's really no need for the 3:00 a.m. feeding. If you can make it to 5:30 a.m., you're essentially there—just start the day then, with breast-feeding or a full bottle, and try to stretch the next feeding as close as you can to 9:00 a.m. in order to make up the time.

Goals: By the End of Week 6

Begin Feeding Time	End Feeding Time	Begin Naptime
6:00 a.m.	6:30 a.m.	7:00 a.m.
9:00 a.m.	9:30 a.m.	10:00 a.m.
12:00 p.m.	12:30 p.m.	1:00 p.m.
3:00 p.m.	3:30 p.m.	4:00 p.m.
6:00 p.m.	6:30 p.m.	7:00 p.m.
9:00 p.m.	9:30 p.m.	10:00 p.m.
12:00 a.m.	12:30 a.m.	

> ### MOTHERLY ADVICE:
> ### DEALING WITH A HARD CRIB MATTRESS
>
> If your baby's crib mattress is unusually firm, give your baby the feeling of softness by inserting a soft blanket underneath the crib sheet to give it a little more cushion. Doing so cannot harm the baby because the padding is underneath the sheet.

Success Story: Becky

Becky and her husband had their first child, A. J., after eleven years of marriage. She works full-time and returned to work when the baby was just seven weeks old.

When my son A. J. was about four weeks old and not sleeping through the night, I was getting a little freaked out. He was waking up every few hours to eat and I was like, "Oh my God, I don't know if I can do this when I go back to work."

Missing sleep was the hardest part. I always had a headache when I was tired. I felt drained, like I couldn't even function. I felt like a walking zombie. My health was going downhill because my eating habits were bad because I was so tired.

My girlfriend, who used The Baby Sleeps Tonight Plan with her twins, recommended that I try it too. Her kids are so good—they sleep and behave so well—so I knew the plan must be wonderful.

Once I got on a schedule I felt things improve very quickly. It was great! Everybody's baby is different and everybody's schedule is different and the plan allows for that based on your family's wake time. If I would have just waited for things to get better on their own, I think I would have been losing my mind by then, because it was just getting worse until it was becoming unbearable.

By the time I went back to work my son was sleeping most of the night. He only needed to have a bottle around midnight and then he slept until 7:00 a.m., so it was already a dramatic difference. And then I kept moving back his last bottle from 11:30 p.m. to 11:00, then to 10:30, then to 10:00, until the time when I actually wanted him to go to bed.

The plan has given us structure. I believe it's helped our marriage. We both were worried because we'd been married for a very long time. We were used to sleeping when we wanted to sleep. We were afraid we'd have no time together. But I think it actually prevented problems since we used the plan so early. Now A. J. sleeps through the night, so we can actually talk to each other and have dinner. My husband and I are both very pleased. I really think it makes the baby happier too. He's always smiling!

Chapter 6

Weeks Seven and Eight

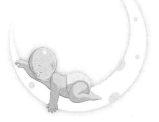

THE ROAD TO EASY STREET

Following The Baby Sleeps Tonight Plan for the last six weeks has helped you to create the day and the night for your baby. All of your little one's needs have been met ahead of time, thereby planting the first seeds of dependability and trust between you and your baby. You should now see that life doesn't have to be a cauldron of chaos! By carefully following this proven schedule, you've already gained a significant amount of order in your household, but it can get even better.

Your goal in weeks seven and eight is to extend the night even longer. In order to do that, we'll have to meet three objectives or stages. You can liken this phase of the plan to a video game; you can't move on to the next stage until you've mastered the one before. A stage is considered mastered when your baby has successfully met the objectives of that stage for at least two nights. Just by making a few simple adaptations we'll have you so close to the "Ultimate Schedule" (chapter 7, eight hours or more of sleep) that everyone will be a winner. Are you ready to play? Let's get started!

Goal #1
Get baby to sleep from 11:30 p.m. to 6:30 a.m.

Weeks 7 and 8, Stage 1 Feeding Times (Every 3½ Hours)

6:00 a.m.	4:30 p.m.
9:30 a.m.	8:00 p.m.
1:00 p.m.	11:30 p.m.

During Stage One, you'll concentrate on extending the night. This means moving the time of the last feeding of the day back to 11:30 p.m., and increasing the wake-time during the day.

In week seven, start the day at 6:00 a.m. and have a thirty-minute feeding as usual. But then extend the wake-time to forty minutes (for a total wake-time of one hour and ten minutes) before putting your baby down for a nap. Then, delay the 9:00 a.m. feeding until 9:30 a.m. and then feed every three and a half hours through the day. Your baby is learning what to expect right now, so we're gradually sneaking in more wake-time during the daylight hours in order to further lengthen the night. Once you've done this successfully for two or three nights straight, you can consider Stage One conquered and move on to the next!

Driven to Distraction

If your baby is having a hard time making it to the next feeding, try to stretch the time to the next scheduled feeding time by redirecting your baby with new activities:

- Dancing with your baby
- Taking your baby outside
- Using positive affirmations
- Watching an educational DVD

Goal #2

Start the day at 6:30 a.m. and introduce a one-hour evening nap.

Weeks 7 and 8, Stage 2 Feeding Times (Every 3½ Hours)

6:30 a.m.	8:30 p.m.
10:00 a.m.	11:30 p.m.
1:30 p.m.	
5:00 p.m.	

Stage Two begins with starting your baby's day a little later, at 6:30 a.m. After the usual thirty-minute feeding, work on keeping your baby up a bit longer, stretching to one hour and twenty minutes total wake-time. Then put baby down for a nap at 7:50.

Another change we'll make in Stage Two is adding a one-hour evening nap from 10:00 p.m. to 11:00 p.m. The necessary step to get your baby sleeping through from 11:30 p.m. to 6:30 a.m. is to wake them at 11:00 p.m. and introduce one more feeding. Why? Because at this age your baby can't quite make it through the night without that extra feeding. You want to make absolutely sure that your baby has been efficiently fed, so that hunger is not a factor in your baby's waking in the middle of the night.

The most challenging thing at this stage is to wake your baby at 11:00 p.m. to feed. Baby will want to sleep, but it's important to complete this step or you will have a middle of the night-waking! The key is to wake him up, change him if he is wet, feed and burp him, and then put him right back to sleep. Once you've established this pattern successfully for two or three nights, then you're ready to move on to the next stage.

Goal #3
Move bedtime to 11:00 p.m. and work toward a 7:00 a.m. wake-up.

Weeks 7 and 8, Stage 3 Feeding Times

6:30 a.m.	8:30 p.m.
10:00 a.m.	11:00 p.m.
1:30 a.m.	
5:00 p.m.	

··· *Note* ···

If you need your wake-time to be something other than 7:00 a.m. you can adapt the schedule accordingly; just remember to keep the same amount of time between feedings.

Stage Three begins by starting your baby's day at 6:30 a.m., but making the night longer by going to bed at 11:00 p.m. Throughout the day, after the usual thirty-minute feeding, work on keeping your baby up a full hour and thirty minutes, then put her down for a nap. The only exception is after the 8:30 p.m. feeding, because you're going to move her 10:00 p.m. nap to 9:30 p.m. Let baby sleep for one hour only, keep her awake until 11:00 p.m., feed her, and put her back to bed at 11:30 p.m.

The way to get your baby sleeping through the night is to make sure that your baby is consuming at least five to eight ounces at this 11:00 p.m. feeding. I recommend making that last feeding a bottle-feeding for a variety of reasons. First, this allows Dad to do a feeding, if he's available, so that Mom can begin her night a little earlier. Second, by using a bottle you can accurately gauge exactly how much your baby has eaten before turning in for this large block of sleep time. Finally, if you're supplementing with formula, those mixtures tend to be a little thicker than breast milk and therefore may keep your baby feeling satisfied longer, thus adding to the likelihood of making it through the night successfully.

But He's Up at 3:00 a.m.!

What do you do if your baby does continue to wake in the middle of the night? Take note of the time that your baby starts to cry and then allow fifteen minutes to pass before entering the room. Sometimes children will quiet down on their own if you don't respond too quickly. If your baby is still awake after fifteen minutes, go into the room and run through the Crying Checklist (page 70), item by item, to make sure that all of her needs have been met. If you've determined that there's no logical reason for the crying, gently pat your baby on the back and use rhythmic shushing to help soothe her, and then go back to bed. At this point, if she is still crying, you have a choice.

You can either let her learn to self-soothe, or you can wait another fifteen minutes before entering the room. If you do go back in, don't stay longer than five minutes. Only allow yourself to go into the room twice throughout the night to quiet the baby. It's very important to pick and choose those times wisely so as not to begin to establish a pattern. (Of course, if your baby is experiencing any kind of illness, stop the plan immediately and return to it as soon as your baby is healthy.)

Good Schedules and Bad Patterns

The Baby Sleeps Tonight Plan is based on creating predictable happiness through the consistent use of a proven schedule. While it's important to stick to the specific details of the plan, it's equally important to avoid establishing your own negative patterns. It's very easy to fall into this trap without even realizing that you're doing it. Patterns are created by responding in the same manner time and time again, thus creating a conditioned response. That repetitive action can quickly become expected by your baby. Fortunately, if you do get yourself into a negative pattern, there are ways to break its hold on you.

Breaking the Pattern of Conditioning

Always be sure to vary the methods that you use to comfort your baby. It's crucially important to use things just occasionally, so that your baby doesn't learn to depend on them. Remember, you want to be the one to establish the patterns, not your baby. Don't always use the same technique. One night you might turn up your sound machine. The next, use rhythmic patting and shushing. The night after that, perhaps playing some rap music softly would help. The strong beat helps to soothe your baby.

When your baby cries, delay your reaction time of response in fifteen-minute increments and soothe him while he's in the crib. You can enter the room before your baby gets into an all-out cry, but then you may run the risk of working him up. Each baby's temperament is different, so you'll have to experiment with different scenarios to know what works best for your particular child.

If you go into the room because your baby is crying, first try to soothe him without picking him up, if you can. The idea is to help your child feel secure while still enabling him to learn to self-comfort.

Remember, it's okay for a baby to make noise. This is part of a baby's growth. It's how you react to your baby that sets the pace. Many times your reactions are more important than your baby's actions. You always want to be part of the solution and not the problem itself.

Recap

Weeks seven and eight can be challenging. The primary goal is to get your baby sleeping from 11:30 p.m. to 6:30 a.m. You do this by gradually moving up the bedtime, increasing the wake-time, and extending the time between feedings. Once you have successfully extended the night, you introduce an evening nap. This will enable you to continue to adjust your baby's schedule. In the end, if your baby is still sleeping when you're ready to wake him for the next feeding, then move on to the next stage.

By the time you hit week nine, you should be ready to move the bedtime feeding to 11:00 p.m. and work toward extending the wake-up time to 7:00 a.m., which is one step closer to the Ultimate Schedule.

Goals: Weeks 7 and 8

STAGE 1

Begin Feeding Time	End Feeding Time	Begin Naptime
6:00 a.m.	6:30 a.m.	7:10 a.m.
9:30 a.m.	10:00 a.m.	10:40 a.m.
1:00 p.m.	1:30 p.m.	2:10 p.m.
4:30 p.m.	5:00 p.m.	5:40 p.m.
8:00 p.m.	8:30 p.m.	9:10 p.m.
11:30 p.m.	12:00 a.m.	

STAGE 2

Begin Feeding Time	End Feeding Time	Begin Naptime
6:30 a.m.	7:00 a.m.	7:50 a.m.
10:00 a.m.	10:30 a.m.	11:20 a.m.
1:30 p.m.	2:00 p.m.	2:50 p.m.
5:00 p.m.	5:30 p.m.	6:20 p.m.
8:30 p.m.	9:00 p.m.	10:00 p.m.–11:00 p.m. 1-Hour Nap
11:30 p.m.	12:00 a.m.	

STAGE 3

Begin Feeding Time	End Feeding Time	Begin Naptime
6:30 a.m.	7:00 a.m.	8:00 a.m.
10:00 a.m.	10:30 a.m.	11:30 a.m.
1:30 p.m.	2:00 p.m.	3:00 p.m.
5:00 p.m.	5:30 p.m.	6:30 p.m.
8:30 p.m.	9:00 p.m.	9:30 p.m.–10:30 p.m. 1-Hour Nap
11:00 p.m.	11:30 p.m.	

MOTHERLY ADVICE: FLEECE SLEEPERS

For a comfortable nighttime sleep, I recommend putting your baby down in a fleece sleeper that has snap enclosures around the legs for easy diaper changing. Fleece sleepers are both comfortable and warm for your little darling so you won't need any additional blankets in the crib.

Success Story: Beth

Beth is the mother of three children who found structure and sanity through the plan. She started The Baby Sleeps Tonight Plan when her second child was seven weeks old.

I'm going to be forty-one years old this year, and I can honestly say that of all the awful things that have happened to me in my life, sleep deprivation ranks right up there. You really can't function when you're sleep-deprived. You can't think for yourself and you really can't think for anybody else. I remember being so tired that I felt like I could just drop the baby because my arms were going to give out on me. It was such extreme exhaustion.

Plus when you're sleep-deprived, depression comes along with that. I don't know anybody who's sleep-deprived who's not down in the dumps. I couldn't see the light at the end of the tunnel with my daughter. I just felt like I was kind of stuck, and tired and frustrated.

In addition to having both a baby and a toddler in the house, I was also working full-time and starting my own business on the side. Talk about overdoing it! I felt like I had a wonderful husband, a beautiful baby, and a sweet little toddler, except I couldn't enjoy it because I was just too tired.

I'm lucky that I do have a very supportive husband, so we were always optimistic, but with a new baby in the house there are so many components that keep the two of you out of sync that your life gets kind of off-track. Suddenly we weren't having conversations about our day like we did before. We didn't go to sleep at the same time and have pillow talk and physical relations like we did before. You're dealing with so many things, including the healing process of your body—it's difficult.

As soon as my husband heard that we could have our baby sleeping through the night he said, "We have to do this!" We were both onboard without any hesitation. At that point I was so sleep deprived it was hard for me to make any decisions. I just needed someone to take the ropes for me and say "Honey, this is what we're doing." This plan was spelling out exactly what I needed to do and I was just like, "Thank God, I finally have an answer!"

I started feeling like I was getting control right away on the plan. We learned from Shari that the baby craves direction, that babies thrive on it and that's where they get their security from. They want to fit into your schedule. Also, with her plan, she has goals, but they were little goals and you would hit them so rapidly that it made you feel like this plan was going to work.

I started to feel hopeful again. I just knew that at some point we were going to be our normal happy family again, with just another sweet little baby, happy and healthy and sleeping through the night like we were.

The hardest part was getting the baby to stay awake when I needed her to stay awake. I remember having to take her clothes on and off, give her a bath, and dance around the house, but I had to do what I had to do to keep this baby awake, because that's what Sergeant Shari told us to do!

With the third baby, my attitude was different right away. We had success before and we knew we would have success again. I was a better mother as a result. I wasn't as tired and it all kind of came together because I knew in advance what we were going to do to conquer the new baby issues. I just felt like I was able to enjoy him instead of freaking out over the process.

I feel like what this plan has done is erase the negative. It's absolutely fool-proof. You can simply enjoy your family, enjoy your life, and enjoy the whole reason that you had a child to begin with.

I always tell new moms about the plan. It doesn't just help you get your baby to sleep; it helps you get your life back. It puts your family on the road to success and happiness. You're telling your baby how to respond, and your baby responds. It's unbelievable! What a miracle!

Chapter 7

Weeks Nine Onward

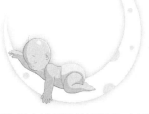

PREDICTABLE HAPPINESS AND BEYOND

Welcome to predictable happiness! During week nine, you'll finally reach a four-hour feeding schedule incorporating five feedings a day, designated naps and wake-times, and, most importantly, eight hours of sleep for you and your family: sleeping through the night!

You have laid the foundation for happiness, and now we'll fine-tune the schedule in order to help you maintain it. We'll work toward the Ultimate Schedule that will lead your child through the toddler years. At this point, we'll introduce a series of designated naps that will give you even more control in planning your life.

As your child ages, you can now expect even longer stretches of sleep, and the Ultimate Schedule is going to help you get there. You should give yourself until week twelve to reach the Ultimate Schedule, but it may happen as early as week ten. It all depends on your baby and your consistency in sticking to the plan.

Goal #1

Get baby on a four-hour feeding schedule with specified naps.

Here's a look at our new schedule:

Weeks 9 Onward, Stage 1 Feeding Times (Every 4 Hours!)

7:00 a.m.	7:00 p.m.
11:00 a.m.	11:00 p.m.
3:00 p.m.	

Weeks 9 Onward, Stage 1 Naptimes

8:45 a.m.	5:15 p.m.–6:15 p.m.
12:45 p.m.	8:30 p.m.–9:30 p.m.

Congratulations! From this stage on, much of this schedule will be written in stone. The 7:00 a.m., 11:00 a.m., and 3:00 p.m. feedings will not change, and the 8:45 a.m. and 12:45 p.m. naps will continue from now on as well.

At this point, it should be becoming clear to you exactly what kind of sleeper your baby is. We're all unique in our makeup. There are some babies that need ten hours of night-time sleep, and others that may need even more. The length of time your baby sleeps on the designated schedule will help you understand your baby's sleep habits. The most important thing is that you put your baby down at the beginning of the naptime. A nap should be at least forty-five minutes long to be considered a nap. After that, you can allow your baby's natural rhythm to determine how much sleep she needs, but make sure it's at least forty-five minutes. (And, of course, if your baby's still asleep at the next feeding time, make sure to wake him up!)

MOTHERLY ADVICE:
PLAN YOUR DAY AROUND NAPS

Take your baby strolling at naptime so that she falls asleep on your walk. When you return home, leave her in the stroller to finish out the nap. You can then take that opportunity to refresh yourself with a nice, hot shower or bath. By the time your baby is ready for the next feeding, you'll be relaxed and raring to go after having some wonderful me-time. You CAN have a life when you plan by the schedule, so take advantage of it. This is predictable happiness...enjoy!

Wake Up! Wake Up!

One challenge you may find on this new schedule is keeping your baby awake until 11:00 p.m. But don't worry—The Baby Sleeps Tonight Plan has all the ingredients for making a recipe for success. Simply refer back to the stimulation techniques outlined in chapter 4 on page 64.

Goal # 2

Once you've achieved the four-hour schedule for at least two days, move the last feeding from 11:00 p.m. to 10:30 p.m.

Weeks 9 Onward, Stage 2 Feeding Times

7:00 a.m.	7:00 p.m.
11:00 a.m.	10:30 p.m.
3:00 p.m.	

Weeks 9 Onward, Stage 2 Naptimes

8:45 a.m.	5:15 p.m.–6:15 p.m.
12:45 p.m.	8:30 p.m.–9:30 p.m.

The only change here is in moving the 11:00 p.m. feeding to 10:30 p.m. You'll keep your baby awake from 9:30 p.m. to 10:30 p.m. (instead of 9:30 p.m. to 11:00 p.m.) and start the last feeding at 10:30 p.m. Stick to the four-hour feeding schedule except for the bedtime feeding.

Make sure you spend only one week maximum at this schedule. Many parents want to stay here because it's a comfortable schedule, but it can be even better, I promise. We're working toward the Ultimate Schedule, but we're not quite there yet.

Goal # 3

Move the 10:30 p.m. feeding to 10:15 p.m.; move the 7:00 p.m. feeding to 6:45 p.m.; and eliminate the 8:30 p.m. nap.

Weeks 9 Onward, Stage 3 Feeding Times

7:00 a.m.	6:45 p.m.
11:00 a.m.	10:15 p.m.
3:00 p.m.	

Weeks 9 Onward, Stage 3 Naptimes

8:45 a.m.	5:15 p.m.–6:15 p.m.
12:45 p.m.	

At this stage, you want to try to keep your baby awake from 6:45 p.m. until 10:15 p.m. without a nap. Granted, this is a quite a long span of time to keep your baby up.

ELIMINATING THE EARLY EVENING NAP

Here's the secret to accomplishing this: put your baby down at 8:30 p.m., but then wake her thirty to forty minutes later. Each night thereafter, continue to decrease the length of the nap by ten minutes until it's gone completely. By the time you get to the Ultimate Schedule, the early evening nap is eliminated.

We're in the home stretch now! Just a few more small adaptations and you will have done in twelve weeks what some families never accomplish.

Goal #4
Start to slowly adjust the last two feedings until you reach the Ultimate Schedule.

Weeks 9 Onward, Stage 4 Feeding Times

7:00 a.m.	6:30 p.m.
11:00 a.m.	10:00 p.m.
3:00 p.m.	

Weeks 9 Onward, Stage 4 Naptimes

8:45 a.m.	5:15 p.m.–6:15 p.m.
12:45 p.m.	

You now need to focus your attention on the 6:30 p.m. and 10:00 p.m. feedings. By adjusting these times you can increase your baby's sleep time to anywhere from ten to twelve hours per night. Your baby will be very receptive to moving the times of these feedings as long as you do it gradually, in small increments of time. Each night, make those last two feedings fifteen minutes earlier until you reach your ultimate goal. Over the span of a few days, your baby will hardly notice the shift, but you will certainly feel it in the morning!

Here's an example of your plan to gradually make those feedings earlier:

STAGE 5

Begin Feeding Time	Designated Naptime
7:00 a.m.	8:45 a.m.
11:00 a.m.	12:45 p.m.
3:00 p.m.	5:00 p.m.–6:00 p.m.
6:15 p.m.	
9:45 p.m.	

STAGE 6

Begin Feeding Time	Designated Naptime
7:00 a.m.	8:45 a.m.
11:00 a.m.	12:45 p.m.
3:00 p.m.	4:45 p.m.–5:45 p.m.
6:00 p.m.	
9:30 p.m.	

MOTHERLY ADVICE: DATE NIGHT

It's important for you and your husband to spend some quality downtime together. Find a good baby-sitter (I will help you with that in chapter 10) and make the decision to go out and enjoy your life together. Why not have some celebratory time rewarding yourselves for different phases and accomplishments you've made on the plan? This really is a group effort, so take some time to pat yourselves on the back and enjoy some much needed leisure time.

Goal #5

Finish adjusting the bedtime to get to the Ultimate Schedule.

The Ultimate Schedule Feeding Times

7:00 a.m. (Breakfast)   6:00 p.m. (Dinner)
11:00 a.m. (Lunch)   9:00 p.m. or earlier (Bedtime)
3:00 p.m. (Snack)

The Ultimate Schedule Naptimes

8:45 a.m. (Morning)
12:45 p.m. (Afternoon)
4:45 p.m. (Catnap)

We just have one more goal to accomplish and you'll be at the Ultimate Schedule. And that goal is the bedtime, which needs to be adjusted by fifteen-minute increments. Make sure you allow a one-hour nap before the dinnertime feeding. At about seven months of age, you'll notice that your baby no longer needs the catnap. When you put your baby down for that nap, she won't want to go to sleep.

As your baby grows, you may certainly adjust the naptimes to 9:00 a.m. and 1:00 p.m., if that works well for you. The nicest thing about The Baby Sleeps Tonight Plan is that you can rest assured that your baby will respond well to these subtle changes because you've worked since day one to instill the security of predictable happiness.

.... *Note* ....

Your final perfected version of the Ultimate Schedule is completely up to you! You can continue to move bedtime up to 9:00 p.m. or earlier; just be sure to wake your baby up at 7:00 a.m. the next day. If your baby isn't waking at 7:00 a.m., keep moving the bedtime until baby wakes on his own.

Now that you have a practical schedule in place and have introduced consistency to your baby, you can fine-tune the schedule to meet your changing needs. You'll have established a pattern perfectly aligned with a healthy eating regimen: five feedings a day. This makes the transition to solid foods much easier, because your baby is already accustomed to eating on a balanced meal-schedule. This feeding schedule will be with your baby all the way through her toddler and childhood years.

Recap

The plan is anchored to your Ultimate Schedule wake-up time, so make every effort to keep that time the same. As you continue with the plan you'll be amazed at the ways your child will grow and flourish, having been given the gifts of order and security. Your child has now learned self-control, knows that she is loved, and anticipates when the next meal is coming.

Goals: Weeks 9 Onward

STAGE 1

Begin Feeding Time	Designated Naptime
7:00 a.m.	8:45 a.m.
11:00 a.m.	12:45 p.m.
3:00 p.m.	**5:15 p.m.–6:15 p.m.**
7:00 p.m.	**8:30 p.m.–9:30 p.m.**
11:00 p.m.	

STAGE 2

Begin Feeding Time	Designated Naptime
7:00 a.m.	8:45 a.m.
11:00 a.m.	12:45 p.m.
3:00 p.m.	**5:15 p.m.–6:15 p.m.**
7:00 p.m.	**8:30 p.m.–9:30 p.m.**
10:30 p.m.	

STAGE 3

Begin Feeding Time	Designated Naptime
7:00 a.m.	8:45 a.m.
11:00 a.m.	12:45 p.m.
3:00 p.m.	**5:15 p.m.–6:15 p.m.**
6:45 p.m.	
10:15 p.m.	

STAGE 4

Begin Feeding Time	Designated Naptime
7:00 a.m.	8:45 a.m.
11:00 a.m.	12:45 p.m.
3:00 p.m.	**5:15 p.m.–6:15 p.m.**
6:30 p.m.	
10:00 p.m.	

Note: Bold indicates times that are changing in weeks 9 onward.

STAGE 5

Begin Feeding Time	Designated Naptime
7:00 a.m.	8:45 a.m.
11:00 a.m.	12:45 p.m.
3:00 p.m.	**5:00 p.m.–6:00 p.m.**
6:15 p.m.	
9:45 p.m.	

STAGE 6

Begin Feeding Time	Designated Naptime
7:00 a.m.	8:45 a.m.
11:00 a.m.	12:45 p.m.
3:00 p.m.	**4:45 p.m.–5:45 p.m.**
6:00 p.m.	
9:30 p.m.	

ULTIMATE SCHEDULE

Begin Feeding Time	Designated Naptime
7:00 a.m.	8:45 a.m.
11:00 a.m.	12:45 p.m.
3:00 p.m.	**4:45 p.m.–5:45 p.m.**
6:00 p.m.	
9:00 p.m. (or earlier)	

Note: Bold indicates times that are changing in weeks 9 onward.

MOTHERLY ADVICE:
TRAVELING WITH YOUR BABY

When traveling, ALWAYS take a sound machine with you for a peaceful nighttime sleep. It allows you to bring the comfort of home with you wherever you go. It's so effective that not only will your baby love it, but you will too. (It can drown out the sound of snoring!)

Success Story: Stacie

Stacie, a successful television anchorwoman, relates her experience with The Baby Sleeps Tonight Plan after the birth of her second child.

I think the reason I'm such a big advocate of the plan is that I didn't use it with my first child and did with the second, and saw such dramatic differences. With my first baby, my son, he was colicky and didn't sleep well and I really did everything at his beck and call. I always felt like I was doing something wrong because he cried all the time. I was feeling like I wasn't a good mom. I didn't know what I was doing. I remember thinking, "You can have a career, you can travel the world, you can meet the president and interview dignitaries, but you can't keep this baby happy." It was a strange place to be in.

But with my daughter I used the plan and really felt like I had everything under control within two weeks. I just stuck to it. I did not deviate from it, and it worked like a charm. She's still a great sleeper. She sleeps through the night and you almost have to wake her up in the morning.

To be a good mom, sleep is such a huge key. You've got all these emotions and you want to be everything to everybody. It's such an exhausting time. It's overwhelming. If you can get the rest and help the baby get his or her rest, then everybody's going to be in a better place.

I think The Baby Sleeps Tonight Plan is a lifesaver for new moms. The demands of being a new parent are so great, if there's anything you can do to make the whole process run a little more smoothly, why wouldn't you? Those initial months are hard. Patterns get established pretty quickly with babies, so I think the sooner you do it, the easier it is. If schedules work for kids all throughout their lives, why shouldn't a schedule work for them as a baby?

Chapter 8

Transitions

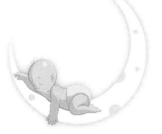

ONE TO GROW ON

You've set The Baby Sleeps Tonight Plan in motion and regained control of your life, and it's exciting to see your little person changing and evolving. Love and predictability are to your child what sunlight and rainwater are to a flower; the more that you shower upon them, the more they will grow.

What's more, now that the whole family is sleeping through the night, you can meet upcoming transitions with a renewed sense of confidence. Your focus at this stage of the game is to keep your baby sleeping through the night by tackling new challenges head-on. As always, the goal of The Baby Sleeps Tonight Plan is to put you one step ahead of what's coming!

You Are What You Eat

Up to this point in your baby's life, she has been able to rely on breast milk or formula for all of her nutritional needs.

Of course, that won't be all she eats for the rest of her life! During the first year, you'll begin to add solid foods to baby's diet and we want to be sure that these additions don't upset the schedule you've worked so hard to establish.

Introducing Cereal

As children grow and expand their diets, it's not uncommon for them to experience some difficulties with digestion. If a certain food upsets your baby, it will in turn upset sleeping patterns. For this reason, it's important to approach feeding solids to your baby in a structured fashion that will allow you to observe your baby's reactions. As with everything on The Baby Sleeps Tonight Plan, there's a method to the madness, so don't worry! I'll walk you through the process step-by-step.

When it's time to make the transition to solid foods you'll be perfectly positioned because the plan already accommodates a healthy eating schedule: breakfast, lunch, and dinner, plus two snacks (which equals five feedings a day, plus allows your baby sleep through the night).

Typically around the four-month mark, your pediatrician will recommend starting rice cereal. Feeding your baby rice cereal for the first time can be quite the experience. The first feeding sessions will be more about getting your baby used to the taste and texture than about actual food intake. As eager as your little one may be to try something new, he or she will probably only get a little bit in at first. This is completely normal.

Part of the reason is because babies have to learn to master their tongue-thrust reflex, which is a forward tongue motion that happens when baby's lips are touched. This natural reflex serves the purpose of helping the baby gain command of breast- and bottle-feeding, but can make eating solid foods more difficult. Many parents mistake this instinctive reaction as a dislike for food. Keep practicing with your baby until he develops the muscle control to take in a mouthful of food and swallow it. Most babies will have figured this out by six months, but until then eating will be a work in progress. Always closely observe your baby to avoid the possibility of choking.

To begin, mix some of the rice cereal with either breast milk or formula until it has a paste-like consistency. You can warm it up if you like, but remember that your baby will grow accustomed to however you're serving it. Seat baby securely in a high chair, and be sure that your baby is sitting upright and not lying down. It's often easiest to begin solids during the early feedings of the day on your current feeding schedule. The first few attempts can possibly cause some gastrointestinal distress, so introducing cereal at an earlier feeding won't interfere with nighttime sleep.

MOTHERLY ADVICE: PLANES, TRAINS, AND AUTOMOBILES

Make eating fun! A great way to make mealtime enjoyable for your baby is to pretend that the spoon is a choo-choo train, an airplane, or a car. Place some food on the spoon and move it around while making the noise of whatever vehicle you've chosen:

- "Open your mouth, the airplane's coming down for a landing!"
- "Choo, choo...Here comes the train into the tunnel!"
- "Vroom, vroom...Open up the garage!"

Your goal is to get your baby eating and trying new foods without objection. Although you may feel foolish doing this, your baby will be having so much fun that mealtime will be a pleasure instead of a chore. In order to avoid creating a conditioned response, guard against doing this every time you feed as your child may come to expect it.

Introducing Baby Food

Since you're still using formula or breast milk, adding baby food is nutrition on top of nutrition. Don't worry about supplying a balanced diet at this point; just focus on getting your baby familiar with variety. This is where your baby's own likes and dislikes come into play, and you can start to gain some knowledge of what your baby enjoys. I always tell my clients that you can recognize the foods your baby prefers by keeping an eye out for the "baby-bird look." Their mouths will be wide open and just waiting for the next morsel to go in! It's important to find your rhythm and not feed too fast; don't let the baby bird lead you—you lead her. You should encourage your baby to eat, but never force her. Every baby will develop his or her own distinctive palate. That's what makes each of us different and unique.

Remember to introduce new foods at the first two feedings of the day. That way you'll have plenty of time to look for any adverse reactions your baby may have. If you introduce a new food before bed and it doesn't agree with your baby, you can be sure that it will disturb his nighttime sleep.

With every new food you introduce, you must watch for possible allergies. Acidic foods can cause reactions too. If, after beginning solids, your baby's sleep patterns suddenly seem disrupted, there's a good chance he may be experiencing some digestive difficulties. Diarrhea or skin eruptions are signs that a certain food might be suspect. In that case, resort back to something that you know your baby tolerates well and make a mental note to reintroduce the suspect food later on. You should always test suspicious foods at least twice before you discard them from the menu entirely. Sometimes children will even outgrow their reactions, so don't be afraid to experiment a little.

It's only natural to want the best for your baby. Consequently, some new mothers choose to make their own baby food using only organic fruits and vegetables. This is certainly an option but make sure that you puree the food smoothly. Swallowing is a challenge for your little one and you don't want to inadvertently create a choking hazard. Although making your own baby food may be a healthier alternative, it's not necessary if your life is too busy. Most of us were fed from traditional baby food jars and somehow we managed to survive. Why place another stress or burden on yourself if you don't have to? There are no hard and fast rules here. The manner in which you feed your baby is strictly your own preference and totally up to you.

As far as introducing types of foods goes, you'll want to start with items that are easily digestible. Remember, a happy tummy equals happy sleep! Here's the way it breaks down:

Grains

Start with grains. Some taste better than others, but oatmeal is a good place to begin. Oatmeal with banana flakes will most likely be well received by your baby. Remember this is your baby's first exposure to different flavors and textures. Your baby's facial expressions and receptiveness to the spoon will indicate which ones are preferred.

Fruits

Once your baby has tried a variety of grains you can begin to introduce fruits. Start with prunes in the morning, as it jump-starts your baby's daily bathroom ritual. Don't worry; prunes are a natural source of fiber but will not cause severe diarrhea. Mixing a spoonful of pureed prunes in with rice cereal will make it a bit sweet and more preferable to your baby. As with all foods, stick with one fruit for a few days before introducing another. Once certain fruits have been successfully tested, then you can begin combining them to create new taste sensations for your baby, if you prefer.

Vegetables

Vegetables are next. Sometimes vegetables are a tough sell to your baby after he has experienced the sweetness of fruits, but allow your baby to try an item for at least a few days before you decide that he doesn't like it. He may just need to grow accustomed to it. As always, don't force, just encourage. Pediatricians often suggest sticking with vegetables of the same color first before moving on to another color. Start with carrots and sweet potatoes, and then move on to peas and green beans. After giving him ample opportunity to see if he likes something, it will become apparent which vegetables your baby prefers.

Meats

Meat is the last thing you'll add to your baby's diet. Make sure all meats are in jars labeled stage one, so that they're finer in texture and easier to swallow. Start with poultry, then move on to beef.

More Foods, Less Milk

Once your baby has mastered all of the food groups, you can start offering combinations of foods at mealtime. If your child is eating a balanced diet of solid food, then don't worry if she's not consuming as much from the bottle. At this stage, shift your feeding emphasis onto solids, and then top off with formula or breast milk. The goal is to have your child totally on solids by one year.

Check with your child's pediatrician about when to drop breast milk or formula. If your child is gaining weight and receiving adequate nutrition, your child's doctor may recommend switching to cow's milk as early as the nine-month mark.

At this time you can begin to introduce a sippy cup as an alternative to the bottle as well. Finding a cup with a longer spout will make it easier for your child to master. Allow her to use the 3:00 p.m. snack-time feeding to learn how to drink from it. Once she has that down, replace the bottle with a sippy cup at all feedings, except the last feeding. For comfort reasons I recommend sticking with the bottle for this night-time feeding. Your child will be making many transitions during this time period and that little bit of familiarity at bedtime will keep her feeling secure and sleeping through the night soundly.

At one year you can begin transitioning away from the bottle, and by fifteen months, the bottle should be gone entirely.

Sweet Nothings

It pays to become aware of the nutritional values of the items that you feed your baby. Know your sugar content! One of the biggest fallacies is that yogurt is great for your baby. Most brands are loaded with sugar. Sugar can cause hyperactivity, irritability, and restless sleep. Become an advocate for your baby and train yourself to check the ingredient lists of the items you purchase. Since sugar can contribute to night-waking, try to eliminate sugar after 3:00 p.m. Not to sugarcoat it, but nothing is sweeter than sleeping through the night!

MOTHERLY ADVICE: THE POWER SHAKE

On the run? You can deliver all the nutritional value of a well-balanced meal inside a bottle by creating a power shake. Combine formula or breast milk with a teaspoon of prunes and two teaspoons of rice cereal. Children love it! These are great to have in reserve for when you can't have a normal, relaxed feeding session.

Night-Waking

Once you've mastered feeding your baby solids and discovered which foods are most likely to disturb his sleep, you may feel as if everything will be smooth sailing from here on in. Unfortunately, the mere nature of life guarantees that other potential sleep hurdles will pop up. Even though your baby has been successfully sleeping through the night for months, he may start experiencing some night-waking. As we've said all along in The Baby Sleeps Tonight Plan, forewarned is forearmed. The sooner you realize what's happening, the sooner you can take measures to correct it and restore blissful sleep. Here's a list of some of the most common causes of night-waking in children as they age, anywhere from six months to two years.

Teething

If you've already gone through the Crying Checklist (page 70) and can't find a reason for the crying, look inside your baby's mouth. She may be cutting a tooth. All children begin teething in their own time, but most commonly, the first tooth appears around six months of age. A complete set of all twenty baby teeth may not be present until your child is two-and-a-half years old.

Teething can be painful for your child. Since she can't verbally express this to you, it's your responsibility to recognize the signs and take measures to relieve her discomfort. Be supportive and encouraging. These are growing pains and won't last forever. Here are some clues to be on the lookout for if you suspect your child might be teething and some helpful tips so your baby can get right back to sleep:

Signs of Teething

- Drooling—This is the textbook, telltale sign for teething. If your baby's chin is constantly wet, odds are a tooth is coming in. Keep a bib handy.

- Diarrhea—The theory is that due to excess drooling, stools pass through the intestines more quickly and take with them more acidic matter. This acidic content can cause diarrhea and result in a painful rash.

- Pain—Watch your baby's reactions. Some children have higher pain tolerances than others. Your baby may gesture to show discomfort by touching his or her face or cheeks.

- White gums—A baby's gums will appear white as the gumline stretches to accommodate the incoming tooth.

- Biting—If the baby chomps down on your knuckle or wants to chew on everything, he may be searching for a way to self-massage his sore gums. Also if he's bottle-feeding and starts gumming the nipple, that's a sign.

- Low-grade fever—Many times a baby who's teething will run a low-grade temperature of up to 100 degrees. If your baby's temperature exceeds 100 degrees, I recommend contacting your pediatrician.

- Irritability—If you notice that your baby's demeanor has changed, this might be an indication of teething.

- Bleeding—Some bleeding is normal as the teeth begin to cut through the gums and is usually short-lived.

Prescription for Teething

If you know your baby is teething, there are several different approaches you can take to help ease the pain.

Gum Massage

I've always found that massaging the baby's gums before bed can be helpful. With clean hands, insert your finger into your baby's mouth and rub the gum-line with a bit of pressure. You may actually be able to feel the hard edge of tooth just underneath the surface. Rubbing your baby's gums will have a soothing effect on your baby and may help the tooth to break through a bit sooner. This is great to do right before bedtime.

MOTHERLY ADVICE:
VIBRATING GUM MASSAGER

There are special teethers that you can buy that look like a rattle but begin to vibrate when the baby bites down on them. The surface is textured so that it provides a soothing sensation for your baby's sore gums. The teether contains a sealed internal battery and creates a massaging action that can help to take the edge off a baby's discomfort.

Numbing Agents

Benzocaine is a numbing medication that can be applied topically to the gums to help ease pain and discomfort. Baby Orajel is a commonly used brand. These medications can be especially helpful just as the tooth is beginning to come in. Make sure that you choose a benzocaine formulation made especially for infants, as adult versions may be too strong for babies. There are even nighttime formulas that seem to work very well.

MOTHERLY ADVICE: FROZEN TOWEL

When your baby is in pain, it can be frustrating for everyone. If you're ready to throw in the towel, do it, literally! Wet a face towel and throw it in the freezer. Once it's partially frozen, pull it out and let your baby chew on it. The cold towel will have a pleasing, numbing effect on your baby's sore gums. Be prepared that they may get a little wet, but most children find this to be very comforting.

Pain Relievers

Giving your baby a dose of pain reliever can also help. Both Tylenol (acetaminophen) and Motrin (ibuprofen) can be effective for relieving your baby's pain. Ibuprofen is an anti-inflammatory and needs to be taken on a full stomach. For this reason, I usually recommend acetaminophen, because you don't have to worry about stomach irritation. You can decide which one works best for your baby. Oral pain relievers can take up to twenty minutes to take effect, so if you know your baby is teething, give her a dose just before the last feeding. If your baby wakes approximately four to six hours later, you'll know that it's worn off and the pain has returned. If so, quietly go into the room and administer another dose. Always remember to check with your pediatrician about proper dosages based on your baby's weight.

.... *Note* ....

Breast-feeding while a baby is teething can be uncomfortable for you because she may want to chomp down. I recommend taking the time to massage your baby's gums before each breast-feeding session. Whatever you do, do not take a break from breast-feeding! It's important to keep your momentum going in order to maintain your milk supply.

Night Terrors

At approximately two years of age, some children may develop night terrors, and this horrifying experience certainly lives up to its name. Night terrors can be extremely scary for the parent as well as the child. Typically, your child will let out a piercing cry in the night, and when you rush to comfort him you may find him sitting upright in bed with his eyes open. While he appears to be awake, he is actually still sleeping. He may be sweating and thrashing about, upset and scared. Don't try to have a conversation or rationalize with him. Gently ease him down into his bed and pat his back until he's sleeping calmly. Comfort him by repeating reassuring phrases such as "You're okay, you're okay."

Night terrors generally occur about two to three hours after the child falls asleep. They differ from nightmares in that your child might not acknowledge your presence while in the middle of a night terror, and afterward he'll have no recollection of the experience. Although a night terror is certainly a frightening experience, there's no medical treatment necessary. Night terrors are thought to be the result of a maturing and overly aroused central nervous system, and children will outgrow them in time.

MOTHERLY ADVICE: MONSTER SPRAY

Around the age of two, many children develop a fear of monsters, especially before bedtime. The best thing you can do to diffuse their fears is to use "monster spray." Get an empty spray bottle, decorate it, and spray the perimeter of the room like a force field. Going through this bedtime ritual will help your child to feel in a position of control.

The Mind/Body/Potty Connection

One of the biggest hindrances to your child sleeping through the night is an immature bladder, so understandably every parent is anxious to see their child make the transition from diapers to the potty. This can occur anywhere between two and three years of age, but every child is different. The key to success is to wait until your child is showing signs of readiness.

Potty-Training Readiness Checklist

- Does your child have the ability to follow simple instructions?
- Is your child interested in watching you go to the bathroom?
- Is your child staying dry for at least two hours at a time?
- Does your child acknowledge when he or she is wet and protest, wanting to be changed?

Children with an older sibling will often show an early interest in potty-training. This is perfectly normal, so allow them to try, but realize that their immature bladders may not be quite up to the task yet. Base your praise on their efforts and not solely on their victories. Potty-training takes time and patience.

When your child shows signs of not wanting her diaper on, you can buy pull-ups. Pull-ups simulate underwear, but have the absorbency of diapers. They can make kids feel like they're becoming a big girl or boy and give them a sense of pride. Some of the more expensive pull-ups come in bright colors and have pictures of your child's favorite cartoon characters on them, but I suggest buying the cheaper, generic ones instead. Remember the idea is to transition your child from the diaper to real underwear, so you don't want her becoming attached to the pull-ups. Also, do not put underwear over pull-ups. Doing so defeats the purpose and teaches your child that it's all right to go potty in her underwear.

Encourage your child to go to the restroom with you, and watch you go to the bathroom. This is called modeling. Children love to mimic what they see. Since you're their main role model, if you're doing it, odds are they'll want to do it too!

Once your child wants to give it a try, I recommend skipping the baby potty and having her use the regular potty from the very beginning. Not only is it psychologically empowering for your child to go directly to a regular toilet but it saves you an unnecessary step. In order to make a real toilet work for your child's size, get a movable potty insert to put on the real toilet. Your child will feel that it's her throne.

Never push your child, only encourage. Allow her to learn at her own pace. Once your child is showing signs of interest and enthusiasm you can use certain reward systems to encourage her progress. We'll highlight the best of these in more detail in chapter 9.

Remember, accidents will happen and you can't expect your child to maintain a perfect potty record. Many will be incapable of going completely accident-free until sometime between four and six years of age. So be patient and never punish your child for a potty-training mishap. There are a number of things you can do to help promote the likelihood of your child staying dry throughout the night (see the following page).

The Stay-Dry-through-the-Night Checklist

- Eliminate liquids after 6:00 p.m.
- Don't give your child fruit juice after 3:00 p.m.
- Make sure your child tries to go to the bathroom before bed.
- Make sure the bathroom is well lit at night with a night-light.

MOTHERLY ADVICE:
POTTY-TRAINING REWARDS

Always strive to keep your mind in fun mode! Children will respond so much more easily to new challenges when you can make a game of it. If your child is potty-training, it can be pretty boring just sitting there waiting for the forces of nature to work their magic, so why not help it along? Make it a fun experience! Have a jar of Fruit Loops cereal nearby and let them throw one in the potty. Instantly you've created a makeshift bull's-eye! Little boys love to aim for them, and girls enjoy it too. Be ready to offer up something special for a job well done, such as stickers or a treat. Giving the child some incentive for learning can be an invaluable tool.

Success Story: Angela

Angela is a psychologist who used The Baby Sleeps Tonight Plan with her twin girls.

With twins it's especially important to have a routine. Basically, I had two babies and they weren't sleeping, I wasn't sleeping, and life was very difficult. I was up with one baby and would finally get that one to sleep, and then the other one would wake up! It just went on and on. I thought to myself, "There's got to be another way!" It was overwhelming and daunting and more than I could handle. I needed help with finding a schedule to balance everything. The Baby Sleeps Tonight Plan was truly a gift and I'm extremely grateful for that.

My husband was very helpful. He didn't resist the scheduling at all and that was great, because that's what we needed to become fully functioning as a family. Once we started the plan, we had everyone sleeping through the night after about two weeks.

I don't see how anyone could be a sane mom without a schedule. I have a friend who's just starting to implement the plan with her baby and, psychologically speaking, I think that will really free her up as a mother. It helps you to find yourself. That was true for me and many of my friends as well. You have to find your courage inside and just do it. This was really very, very powerful for me.

I'm a clinical psychologist and from that perspective I think the plan helps create predictability and consistency. You know where you're going. It brings a sense of security to the child and I think that's a huge gift. It's a win-win situation for everyone.

For those women out there looking for support, this is it.

This plan was lifesaving for me and my family in those early days. It got me on a fabulous path with my girls with regards to creating boundaries and expectations. I feel incredibly blessed to have had it. It's very empowering, and through it I was able to help myself, my girls, and my family!

Chapter 9

Growing Up

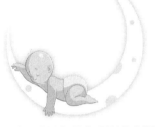

FIFTEEN MONTHS TO TWO YEARS OLD

With The Baby Sleeps Tonight Plan, you have instilled boundaries and limits with regards to eating and sleeping, and the rewards have been significant. Now, the household structure that you've established is more important than ever. In order to maintain the schedule that you've created, and keep your child sleeping through the night, you must strive to balance your child's freedom within the confines of the plan.

As your child becomes more autonomous and independent, she will need your special guidance to keep her both physically safe and emotionally secure. You'll need to be clear and consistent about what's acceptable and what's not. As a parent, the lessons you teach your children will groom them into responsible people who can think for themselves and make good choices. The Baby Sleeps Tonight Plan will make sure of it!

How to Bridge the Nap Gap

The biggest sleep-related change that will happen in this time period is the elimination of the 8:45 a.m. morning nap. Anywhere from fifteen to eighteen months you may notice that when you put your child down for the first nap, he won't seem tired and will begin to resist sleep. This is perfectly normal at this stage. Now is the time to begin to adapt the Ultimate Schedule we outlined in chapter 7 in order to move to just one nap.

To eliminate the morning nap, based on a 7:00 a.m. wake-time, begin by delaying the nap by forty-five minutes to start at 9:30 a.m.; however, still wake your child at 11:00 a.m. to eat. Over the next few weeks, push the nap forward even more, to 10:00 a.m. and then to 10:30 a.m., but continue to wake him at the 11:00 a.m. feeding. The afternoon nap will stay the same at 12:45 p.m., until you have eliminated the morning nap.

Begin Naptime	Feeding Time	Begin Naptime
9:30 a.m.	11:00 a.m.	12:45 p.m.
10:00 a.m.	11:00 a.m.	12:45 p.m.
10:30 a.m.	11:00 a.m.	12:45 p.m.
Eliminated	11:00 a.m.	12:00 p.m.

Your objective is to gradually eliminate the morning nap altogether by keeping your child up through the 11:00 a.m.

lunchtime feeding. All children will do this at their own pace but the eventual goal is to begin the afternoon nap around noon. By the age of eighteen months, most children will have settled into this new napping schedule. At that point, put your child down for a nap and let him sleep as long as is natural for him, making sure that he doesn't sleep past 3:00 p.m. As your child gets older, you can adjust the nap to start at 1:00 p.m. Most children will stay on this schedule, with one long nap, up until approximately three years of age.

Around the preschool years, your child's need for sleep will naturally decrease. At this point I recommend encouraging your child to take a "rest-time," which may not involve sleeping but instead reading or simply quiet time.

Safety

A happy family is life's most precious gift, and one of your jobs as a parent is to protect that happiness by keeping everyone safe. Although this may sound like a difficult task, it's really just an extension of what you've been doing all along—instilling boundaries and limits.

Play Yards

The use of play yards can be beneficial if used wisely. Play yards can be an effective tool for both naptime, wake-time, and nights away from home. If you like the security provided by keeping your child contained in an enclosed area, then I recommend using it from the very beginning. Make play-yard-time a regular part of your child's day and refer to it as her "special place." Be sure to keep your terminology positive regarding the play yard so that she'll see using it as a positive experience. Consistency is the key to your child accepting the play yard without resistance. If you only use it occasionally, she won't want to be there. Play yards can be a useful tool for when you need to be away from your child momentarily without worry.

Crib Safety

Once your child has the ability to stand, I recommend lowering the crib mattress to its lowest setting in order to avoid accidents. If your little person can put his elbows on top of the rails, then it won't be long before he's lifting himself up and out of there! Keeping the crib low to the ground will help him to avoid falls.

Also, when your child is mobile and still in a crib, it's a good idea to supply him with a wake-up activity. You don't want him attempting to scale the sides of the crib before you can get there. Place one or two safe items in the crib with the child so that he'll have something to occupy himself with in the morning. Make sure that anything you put in the crib is age-appropriate and not a hazard to your child. Explain that he is to wait in the crib until Mom and Dad get there. You can do this at naptime as well. This will help him to become independent and learn to exercise self-control.

Baby-Proofing

You must always keep an eye on children who are mobile. Never assume that they're safe. Before your child is allowed to roam freely, do a thorough check of your home, addressing any safety concerns. If you'd like to hire a professional, many companies specialize in baby-proofing. They'll come to your house with all the necessary safety items to keep your child out of harm's way. There are many potential danger areas lurking in your home that you might not be aware of. Here are some to watch for:

- **Electrical outlets**—There are several different types of outlet covers that you can buy that protect little hands from danger.
- **Blind cords**—Although easily overlooked, blind cords can present the danger of strangulation to your child. The loop in the cord can function as a noose. I recommend either cutting them into two single pieces, or affixing the cord high on the wall out of the reach of your child.
- **Rugs**—Rugs that aren't secured to the floor can cause a new walker to trip and fall.
- **Drawers, cabinets, and closets**—Little hands love to explore so keep areas that are off-limits secured with child safety locks. These locks keep your child away from dangers such as glassware, knives, and household chemicals.
- **Table edges**—Even the sharp edges of a table can be a danger to an unsteady child. I recommend buying special rubber backing to apply temporarily to avoid possible injuries.

- **Doors**—Children learn by watching you and will learn to open doors in no time. Install special safety handles that prevent doors from being opened by little hands. Be sure to apply them to all doors, especially the ones that lead outside.
- **Windows**—Secure all windows with safety latches, especially on the second floor.
- **Electrical cords**—Keep all electrical cords out of reach or encased in plastic tubing to avoid both electrocution and strangulation risks.
- **Stairs**—Make sure stairs are gated off to avoid potentially dangerous falls.
- **Household cleaners**—Children are notorious for putting everything in their mouths, so it's crucially important to scan the house for potentially poisonous items. Any household cleaners should be stored out of the reach of children. Many other items, such as mouthwash, may pose a danger to your child as well.
- **Pesticides**—The use of pesticides inside and outside the home can pose a threat to both children and animals. Many fertilizers can also be harmful. Explore herbal alternatives as a replacement to those that may be potentially dangerous.
- **Yard landscaping**—A beautiful yard is wonderful, but not at the expense of your child. Be aware that some plants and flowers in your yard may be poisonous if consumed. Become educated about the toxicity hazards of any items used in your landscaping.

- **Locks**—Consider putting locks on toilets, appliances, and fireplaces to avoid mishaps.
- **Furniture**—Make sure that furniture and lamps are securely fastened to the floor.

.... *Note* ....

Even though you may have taken every measure to protect your child, you must still be prepared for any potential problems that may arise. Always have a list of emergency numbers by the telephone and keep a container of syrup of ipecac handy to induce vomiting in case your child does consume something that is potentially dangerous. Contact your local poison control for additional support if needed.

From a Crib to a Bed

If you're like most parents, you might prefer to keep your child in a crib for as long as possible, because she's somewhat contained and you can be better assured of her safety. However, when the time comes for your child to make the transition to a bed, you'll know it. Many times her physical skills have long surpassed the effectiveness of guardrails and she'll learn to scale them as naturally as a monkey climbs a tree! Although it might mean more work for you, moving her to a bed is an important part of her emotional growth and encourages a sense of freedom and independence.

The age of twenty months is an ideal time to make this transition for many reasons. Not only is your child mobile, but many families plan the birth of a second child around this time frame as well. The new baby can then take over the crib, and you can use this opportunity to build self-esteem in the older child by making her feel as if she's getting something special by moving to her own bed.

The key to a successful transition to a bed is to make sure that both the room and the child are secure. It's vitally important that the room is baby-proofed, due to your child's newfound mobility. Limit the amount of things in the room. Keep it simple. Be sure to rid the room of any potential hazards.

Remember that this room, no matter how special you make it, is a new environment for your child and it will take some getting used to. Keeping a sense of familiarity can be very comforting for your little one. Bring the magic of the sound soother along. Not only will it help to ease any fears that your child may have, but it can help to drown out other noises in the house as well. Also, I recommend using objects that your child already loves to help her make the transition from a crib to a bed. Allow her to take along favorite stuffed animals, dolls, or blankets from the crib to the bed as long as they don't pose a hazard.

Crib Breakdown Party

Even though your child may seem eager to be rid of the crib, this has been his domain for almost two years, so don't take it down without his knowledge. Big changes can cause emotional stress for your child, so it's much better to allow him to participate in taking apart or moving the crib. Why not make this milestone a celebration? Have a crib breakdown party with balloons and special treats. Play some of your child's favorite music and make a really big deal out of it. Make it a fun experience, while placing the emphasis on gaining something, rather than losing something. If you'll be using the crib for a new baby and can't move it to another room, then always change the look of the room to avoid jealousy or possessiveness on the part of the older child. Even if you re-created a mini-version of Disney World for your older child, you can be sure that he won't take well to seeing the new baby taking over his old stomping ground.

Selecting a New Bed

When selecting a new bed for your child it pays to think about the future. Toddler beds are close to the floor and better suited for the size of your little one, but you'll probably need to replace it with something larger in a few short years. A full-sized bed is fine for a young child as long as it's covered on all sides by guardrails or up against a wall. Letting your child take part in the selection of the new bed will help to foster a sense of ownership. Narrow the field of choices but then let him make the final decision. Also let him choose the decorating style of the new room. Keeping your child involved in the process, right down to making the bed for the first time, will help him take pride in his new surroundings.

The First Night in the New Room

The first night in her new "big kid" room is a milestone for your child. It's important to do things right from the very beginning. Prepare her ahead of time by letting her know that this is the first step to becoming a big girl (or boy). Try using a baby gate instead of closing the bedroom door so that your child doesn't feel so isolated. Communicate to her that this is her safety gate. Have her decorate it and make it her own accomplishment. This gate will give her a sense of security within her new environment and create a safe boundary. It will give you peace of mind not to have her mobile throughout your home during naptime and sleep time.

Read her a bedtime story either seated in a chair or on the floor. The idea is to create a cuddle spot for you and your child other than the bed. After your bedtime ritual, let her get into the bed, but do not lie with your child. Remember, the bed is for sleeping! Have a night-light or dimly lit lamp in the room, and turn on your child's sound soother or some soft music. Tuck her in and let her know you'll come back in five minutes to check on her. Take this as a vow and make sure that you do indeed come back as promised. You're building trust with your child and diffusing any fears of abandonment. This practice will heighten her sense of security and self-control. Limit coming back to only twice per night. If the first few nights are very challenging and you need to rub your child's back, that's fine. Worst-case scenario, Mom or Dad may lie down on the floor, but NEVER in the bed! (If you do, you'll always have to do that.) Your job is to help her welcome this new stage of her life as independently as possible. It will understandably take a few nights for her to become accustomed to her new sleeping arrangements, so be patient.

Because your child is now mobile and can theoretically get out of bed whenever he wants to, I suggest giving him some guidelines. First, get a digital clock and communicate what time you'll be back to get him. Since children can't comprehend time at this age, you'll have to play a matching game of sorts. For example, if 7:00 a.m. is the time to get up, then print out and tape 7:00 above the digital display on the clock. Your child will learn to look for those numbers as an indicator of when you'll be there to get her. I also recommend giving him a wake-up activity. If he wakes earlier than anticipated, have a book set aside that he can read until you get there.

MOTHERLY ADVICE: MOMMY OR DADDY DOLL

Changing your child's routine by moving her to a new room can temporarily bring up some attachment issues. It's perfectly normal that she might want to run to you in the night, but it's important to reinforce her boundaries by explaining that everyone has his or her own space. In order to help ease the separation anxiety, purchase a mommy or daddy doll. Take your child shopping and have her choose a doll that represents Mommy or Daddy. The doll becomes a nighttime substitute for you. Put the doll in bed with your child and tell her to hold it tight whenever she misses you. Reassure her that there's nothing to be frightened of, and that the doll will watch over her and protect her. You might even want to spray your perfume or cologne on the doll so that it will smell like you. This can also have a calming effect on your child.

Eliminate the Negative

Around this time, children naturally begin to assert their newfound sense of independence by pushing the envelope a bit. When your child is faced with a major change like moving to his own room, he may experience conflicting emotions and frustrations that he doesn't know how to control or express and may become defiant about sticking to the plan.

Addressing "No"

There's power in the word "no" and somehow children just seem to know it! Many children will try to exercise their independence this way. The most important thing you can do when dealing with negative behavior is to keep your own reaction in check, and NEVER compromise the schedule. If you give in to a tantrum, or get angry and raise your voice, it only escalates the negative behavior. It's best to remain calm at all times.

Through your words and your tone you are sending a very powerful message. Strength comes across much better by being calm rather than yelling. You show that you're in control when you don't allow yourself to be shaken by bad behavior. There's no reason to bargain or cajole; just simply and clearly state your displeasure. Begin by taking three deep breaths and looking your child straight in the eye. Lower the pitch of your voice and firmly say, "We don't do that."

Although the "no" stage can be very trying for parents, this behavior is perfectly normal and speaks to your child's growing security and independence. He is working to develop the confidence that will be needed as he ventures out into the world of making friends and starting school. Your challenge is to guide him into finding the balance between confidence and defiance while keeping him on a healthy and manageable schedule.

MOTHERLY ADVICE:
HANDLING TANTRUMS

Growing up isn't easy. It's no wonder that children sometimes feel the need to express their frustration. Instead of
always trying to talk your child out of his negative feelings,
why not help him release them? A great tool for this is the
"pounding pillow." If your child starts to hit, explain that
it's not acceptable to hit other people but he can pound
on the pillow instead. It's crucial that children have physical outlets to release pent-up aggressions. If you notice
his frustrations increasing, try to include more outdoor
play into your schedule. Running, jumping, and climbing
are great ways to eliminate stress in a healthy manner.
Just as you do, teach your child to take three deep breaths
in order to diffuse his or her anger.

Accentuate the Positive

When your child makes the transition to a bed, this is the
perfect time to begin using rewards as incentives for good
behavior. It brings fun and happiness into the household
and allows you to control your child in ways other than
force of will. This is a busy time in your little person's life
and it never hurts to offer some incentive for all her hard
work. If your child shows the restraint to stay in bed in the

mornings, instead of traipsing all over the house, acknowledge her effort! There are a couple of excellent reward techniques that will work wonders for keeping your child motivated to stay on the schedule.

Using Star Charts

A star chart is a board that outlines your child's top duties. This wonderful reward system is perfect for children as young as two years old. Since your child can't read yet, use pictures to depict each job, leaving space beside them for each day of the week. A typical chart might have pictures of sleeping in a bed, a toothbrush and toothpaste, combed hair, a potty, and toys. Each picture represents something that your child is expected to do each day. Whenever your child accomplishes that goal, she gets to place a big, shiny star next to that day. The stars come in a variety of different colors and children love to see how many shiny stars they can accumulate. At the end of the week, if she has all the stars on her chart, then she has earned a reward. Make a celebration of it! As your child gets older you can change and adjust the responsibilities on the chart. Kids love having a visual reminder of their accomplishments; it encourages them to help out, and it makes learning fun.

Treasure Chest

Who doesn't love to indulge in the fantasy of digging through a big treasure chest? To a child, there's nothing better than a surprise! When your little person exhibits good behavior and starts to act in responsible ways, you can reinforce that behavior by offering a trip to the treasure box. Start by creating a box whose sheer presence will instill excitement in your child. Allow him to decorate it with markers and paint, and then top it all off with some shiny stickers! Explain to your child that you'll fill the box with all sorts of toys, treats, and goodies, but it's reserved for those special moments when his good deeds need to be rewarded. Make sure that your child knows that only YOU will have access to the box. Seeing this beautiful box, full of surprises, will give him the incentive to do more good things. In order to keep the box special though, you'll need to limit its use to no more than two or three times a week. The treasure chest can be especially effective when you "catch" your child doing good out of the blue. For example, if you see him willingly share with another child, a trip to the treasure chest would be a great way to let him know that you're proud of him and reinforce that good behavior!

When filling this special container, remember that everything is exciting and new to a child. The gifts don't have to be elaborate. Perhaps you could include coupons for a movie rental or an ice cream cone. Stickers and treats always seem to go over well. Not only is this practice fun for your child, but it also demonstrates to him that you notice the good as well as the bad. All children crave attention.

The goal is to create a child who learns to seek out attention in positive ways as opposed to grabbing the limelight through negative behavior. Rewards offer a simple and fun way to do that!

Attachment Items

Many children find their security early in life from attachment items, such as a favorite blanket or a pacifier. These items can initially be helpful to your child as they aid in her feelings of independence and control. Many children find it much easier to go to sleep while cuddling their favorite stuffed animal for comfort. As your child ages, however, you can lessen her dependence on these objects by using them only occasionally. For example, much of the appeal of a binky is the sucking satisfaction the child receives. In order to lessen the enjoyment, cut the tip off of the pacifier. Be prepared for your child's inevitable dissatisfaction by providing her with a new transitional item. Hand her a soft blanket and instruct her to rub the corner of it on her face for comfort. Most children will feel soothed by the blanket's softness. The idea here is to focus on trading up. Carrying around a blanket is more acceptable than sucking on a binky. Instead of taking away attachment items cold-turkey, gradually move them on to more acceptable forms of comfort. Eventually these items will begin to lose their appeal and your child will be sleeping soundly and securely without them.

Family Bedtime Rituals

As your child grows, the way you approach bedtime will naturally change and evolve. Wind-down time is very important. At least thirty minutes before bedtime you should cease all stimulating activity. This can be difficult because many parents don't even get home from work until right before their child goes to bed. This can be counterproductive, because the child then becomes too excited to sleep. If at all possible, try to allow yourself thirty minutes with your child before the bedtime ritual. Keep it low-key. No roughhousing or physical play should be allowed.

Never tell your child to "go to bed." Watch your wording. If your child is over-stimulated or having sleep issues, this can seem like a command and cause anxiety. At naptime, call it "rest time." At bedtime, call it "nite nite time." Children will respond better when you soften the edges a bit and avoid being too direct.

Establishing some family bedtime rituals will help your child's sleep habits immensely. It gives him something to look forward to and makes bedtime less of a battle. More importantly, it sets aside a specific time every day for you to connect as a family. Here are a couple of my favorite family bedtime rituals:

Family Circle

Parents, siblings, and baby sit on the floor in a circle and everyone gets the opportunity to talk about the highs and lows of the day. If baby can't talk yet, then you speak for her. Express your feelings. What made you happy or sad? This activity allows the child to know that Mom and Dad have feelings too, and that both good and bad things can happen to everyone. Continuing this open communication helps the family to become more connected. You can end the evening with prayers or positive affirmations and your plans for tomorrow.

Question Chair

Open communication in a family makes each member feel valued. Get a special chair that's deemed the "question chair." Allow each child to sit in the chair and ask a question about anything. It's best to limit the questions to about four per night. Sitting in the chair makes that person the center of attention and allows them to be heard. Children love it!

MOTHERLY ADVICE: FLASHLIGHT

Allowing your two-year-old to take her very own flashlight to bed with her is a great idea! It gives her a sense of control over the darkness, helps to soothe fears, and allows her to read after the lights are out. Let there be light!

More Wind-down Suggestions

You can help your child get ready for a good night's sleep by implementing activities to encourage relaxation. Some children find a warm bath calming. Soft music at bedtime is also very soothing. Another wonderful activity is reading to your child. This is a great way for your little one to wind-down while sharing some quality one-on-one time with a parent. Give him a choice of what books he wants to read, but be sure to limit to no more than two books per night. As children get older they often attempt to use this as a delay tactic. As the parent, create boundaries and strive to find a happy balance.

If your child communicates that he's not tired, continue to put him to bed at the scheduled time, but suggest that he read a book or listen to some music until he's sleepy. Audio books can be very effective in this instance as well. Before leaving the room, give your child a hug and a kiss, and tell him to think happy thoughts. If your child feels more comfortable with the lights on, then allow him to leave them on (you can always turn them off later).

Success Story: Jodi

Jodi is a working mom who used The Baby Sleeps Tonight Plan for both of her children.

I don't know how I would have lived without The Baby Sleeps Tonight Plan. I run a personal concierge service so I had to have a schedule or I wouldn't have been able to function. And I think it's the best thing for your kids. I really do. You're giving them structure and a sense of responsibility at a young age that they can take with them later.

My first baby was a preemie. He came eight weeks early and had to be in the neonatal unit for the first five weeks of his life. The nurses actually started him on a three-hour schedule that we then adjusted to our time frame. It helped ease any questions about whether a schedule was the right thing to do. If the neonatal unit was doing it, I thought, it must be a good idea.

My husband was amazing. He took time off work to be involved. We discussed this beforehand, because we were sharing feeding times and knew we both needed to be onboard. That was a huge, important part for us.

I have so many friends with kids who haven't used the plan, and our lives are so much easier! We know from 1:00 to 3:00 p.m. our kids are going to nap. There's an expectation. Everybody knows what we're doing and when we're doing it. It's tremendous! It gives you a life.

Chapter 10

When You're Not in Charge of Baby's Schedule

hether it's to return to work, run errands, or just take a much-needed break, eventually you'll have to entrust the care of your little person to someone else. Making the decision of whom to leave your child with can leave you feeling vulnerable and uneasy. Although it may not be pleasant, these reactions are completely normal. It's a mother's natural instinct to be protective of her children. This is yet another powerful expression of the connection between parent and child.

It's important to recognize that this new caregiver will be instrumental in maintaining the schedule that you've spent the last few weeks establishing. The caregiver's efforts can make it or break it. Even though your child may be sleeping through the night, he can quickly lose that if someone isn't there to reinforce all your hard work. Be very diligent about communicating all aspects of The Baby Sleeps Tonight Plan to potential applicants ahead of time to make sure that they're receptive to it. I would advise them to read this book so that they better understand the system and the positive rewards that are gained by it.

Whatever your circumstances, whether you need child care or just choose to have it, don't feel guilty. Opening up your child's life to other people and circumstances will enable her to grow and have experiences that you might not have been able to provide. This added dimension will add richness to your child's life. Although it may be nerve-racking, as long as you make good choices regarding this new caretaker, the experience will be a positive one for both you and your baby.

In addition to the obvious safety concerns you may have, learning to share the love and trust of your child can be equally as hard. For a new mom, who has been inseparable from her baby for months, this can be rather traumatic. Not only has this baby been the biggest part of your life, but also a part of you, so understandably letting go can be difficult. It's important to remember that love knows no boundaries. This new caretaker will develop a bond with your child, and vice versa, but this new relationship will in no way lessen the connection that you and your child share. The more love and kindness your baby receives, the more likely your child is to grow into a secure, well-adjusted, and flourishing adult.

In order for things to go smoothly, it's crucially important that you're comfortable with the person you choose. I suggest that you start your search even before the baby is born. Take some time to assess your own personal situation with regards to wants and needs, and research what resources are available to you locally. In addition to searching the Internet, word-of-mouth referrals can be exceptionally helpful. Ask your friends, pediatrician, and OB/GYN if there's anyone that they recommend. Also visit baby play places, such as a park or a library, and ask around. Finding someone whose great reputation precedes him or her will go a long way toward alleviating your anxiety.

Choosing a Caregiver

Depending on your specific situation, there are several different childcare options that are available to you. You'll have to weigh the pros and cons between a traditional day care establishment, an in-home caregiver, and a nanny to decide which is better suited to your lifestyle. I always recommend first observing possible candidates with your baby before making any long-term commitments. Doing so will increase your comfort level tremendously. Remember, although your rapport with this person is important, this is not your friend. Ultimately, you will be this person's employer and your baby's best interest has to be your primary concern. You're putting your baby's well-being in someone else's hands, literally, and it's your parental responsibility to ask the right questions to make sure that this person is qualified to do the job. Once you're sure the answer is yes, then you can open your heart to this individual and allow him or her to become another link in the strong chain you've created.

To start your search, there are certain items that you must address, regardless of which type of caregiver you choose.

Proximity to Your Home

As parents, we would go to the ends of the earth to ensure our children's safety. Fortunately, odds are you won't have to. Finding a caregiver close to your home or work will be beneficial to you in many ways. First, there's always something comforting about knowing that your child isn't that far away from you. Second, the less travel time you have to schedule into your day, the more time there is for enjoyment and pleasurable activities with your family. Remember, The Baby Sleeps Tonight Plan is about creating predictable happiness, so we're always searching for ways to simplify your life.

First Impressions Count

Never discard your immediate impression of someone. Again, this may be your mother's intuition talking. Of course, it would be wise to look for someone who presents herself in a professional manner, tends her own personal hygiene (check out those fingernails), as well as keeps a clean establishment. Go with your "gut" on this one. If something just doesn't feel right, then it probably isn't. Move on to the next candidate on your list.

CPR Certification

Just as you and your partner prepared for the baby by becoming CPR-certified, so should your caregiver. Any licensed child-care professional should automatically be CPR-certified, but never leave the details to chance. Always ask them specifically. Hopefully your child will never need their expertise in this area, but it's better to be safe than sorry.

Other Qualifications and Certifications

In fact, state and county licensing agencies will require caregivers to meet several qualifications before allowing them to accept children. It would be a good idea to contact your local Department of Child Care Regulation and familiarize yourself with their criteria. Some caregivers may even exceed the basic requirements set by the state, but you won't realize it if you don't do your homework. Being knowledgeable is always a plus.

Approach to Discipline

This is important because you can't assume that everyone agrees on the proper way to discipline a child. Sooner or later, even your "little angel" will need a guiding hand. How will the caregiver address that? People who have made it their business to care for children will have a definitive answer to this question. Your job is to decide whether you personally agree with their tactics or not. You can learn a lot about the temperament of your caregiver by the answer you receive to this question, so be sure to address this issue ahead of time.

Day-Care Questionnaire

There are definite pros and cons to every situation, and choosing a traditional day-care establishment for your child is no different. On the plus side, these institutions are held to a very high standard by state and county authorities. They are made to meet rigorous criteria and are subject to spot inspections. Finding one that has been in business for a considerable amount of time would indicate that they have a good, working knowledge of this.

For an older child, day care can be a wonderful socialization tool. This will be your child's first experiences with sharing and playing with other children, and the activities in day-care centers are generally well structured. On the other hand, if you're taking your infant to a day care, I would certainly find out what the "child-to-caregiver ratio" is. Younger children will need more care and you'll want to make sure that the establishment is able to provide that. Following are some important questions you should ask:

- Will you be able to adhere to The Baby Sleeps Tonight Plan?
- How many children are there in a classroom?
- Which caregivers will be tending to my child?
- What are your emergency procedures?

- What sanitizing methods do you use?
- Are there any late-pick-up fees?
- What holidays are you closed for?
- What's your policy regarding sick children?
- Is there a religious preference or faith-based curriculum at your facility?

MOTHERLY ADVICE: DROP IN TO CHECK UP!

A good way to ease your mind and build trust is to show up unannounced. I believe it's in the best interest of your child for you to stop by occasionally and see if they're actually adhering to the plan. If the day care or caregiver doesn't seem happy to see you stopping by unexpectedly, that may be a red flag. Again, the well-being of your child is your number-one concern, so if dropping by once in a while helps to make you feel more comfortable, then so be it!

In-Home Caregiver Questionnaire

Private-home day cares have become a popular option recently. The caregivers are licensed by the county to keep a certain number of children in their home. Typically, they will only have five to ten children that they watch during the day. They too are held to strict guidelines and spot inspections by childcare authorities. This sort of arrangement often works well for infants because they're generally able to receive a bit more one-on-one attention. Also, it's easier for this type of caregiver to work in The Baby Sleeps Tonight Plan since they're not trying to adhere to the rigorously structured day of a traditional day-care establishment. With an in-home caregiver you'll want to ask the following:

- Can you adhere to The Baby Sleeps Tonight schedule?
- Can I take a tour of your home?
- Can I see your childcare license?
- Who are the other children that attend and what are their ages?
- How often are the kids sick?
- What happens if my child gets sick?
- What play resources are available?
- Do you keep daily documentation of the child's activities?
- Are meals provided? If so, are the meals balanced? What types of foods are being fed?
- How do you sanitize? Do you use rubber gloves when changing diapers?
- Are you certified for nighttime care as well?
- Is there any flexibility in your hours, or are you strict about drop-off and pick-up times?
- Do I pay for the entire week or just the amount of time used?

MOTHERLY ADVICE: MEMENTOS

To help ease separation anxiety, you can leave a special memento for your child to discover when he or she is away from you. I recommend placing a photo of Mom and Dad in your child's lunch box along with a note with encouraging words such as, "Love you," "You're the best," or "Have a great day." This will keep your child connected to you even when he or she is far away.

Nanny Questionnaire

If you're considering hiring a nanny, you must realize that this person will not only be an employee but an extended member of your family. There are several good nanny agencies out there, but you can find great nannies in a number of ways. You can ask for referrals from trusted friends or use online resources such as Craigslist, but ALWAYS run a background check on any individual that you are considering choosing.

If you decide to use a nanny agency, their fee structures vary. Some will charge you one lump sum, and others charge on a "temporary to permanent" basis. In the latter scenario, the agency will handle payments until you decide if you want to keep the nanny permanently. This sort of situation allows the luxury of becoming comfortable with your nanny before making a definite commitment, but you will pay a premium for this. If using a nanny agency, I suggest being as specific as you can about what you're looking for in a nanny. Let them screen the applicants and limit yourself to only interviewing those that meet your criteria. Taking the time to make a list of the ideal candidate's characteristics beforehand will save you time, money, and headaches.

Contacting local colleges and universities can sometimes be a great resource when searching for a nanny. Many times, someone working toward a degree in early childhood education will be interested in employment as a part-time or full-time nanny. This can be a wonderful arrangement for both of you; they get much-needed work experience, and you can usually negotiate a more reasonable price. The one downside to this pairing is that a student will probably only be with you for the short-term. If you know you want someone long-term, this might not be the ideal choice for you, because your child will inevitably develop a bond with this person.

When interviewing potential nannies, I suggest asking them if they prefer a schedule for a child or feeding-on-demand, even before you let them know your preference. Many times people will say what they think you want to hear. It's always nice to know how they truthfully feel about the topic before telling them about The Baby Sleeps Tonight Plan. Also you should strive to be clear about your own expectations. In addition to everything covered in the plan, if you expect the caregiver to bathe your baby, take him for walks, and participate in his playtime, tell him or her that! Other important questions follow:

- Where have you worked before?
- How long have you been with this person? (Check all references.)
- Why did you leave your last job?
- Would you be willing to travel with us and share a room with the baby?
- Do you have prior experience with newborns? What ages were the children you cared for?
- Do you have a driver's license? Will you be able to do a carpool in the future? Run errands?
- What is your cleaning experience? What supplies do you use?
- Will you do laundry?
- Do you like to cook? If necessary, will you be able to prepare a dinner?
- Are there things you like to eat during the day? Do you have any special needs?
- Do you have a cell phone?
- What would you prefer not to do? (Don't find out by chance.)
- Do you love children? Do you have any of your own?
- Do you smoke?
- What are your salary requirements? What are your benefits requirements? (Sick leave/vacation/Social Security)

- Are you bilingual? Will you speak/teach in English or your native language?
- What are your personal strengths and weaknesses?

> ## MOTHERLY ADVICE:
> ## THE COMFORT OF HOME
>
> If your child is having any sleep related issues at the day care, why not take along the sound soother? Hearing the sound that your baby has grown accustomed to will help to make the transition easier. Anytime you go to a new place, taking along familiar sounds, smells, and sensory-related objects will help you to comfort your child.

The Nanny-Cam Debate

I recently had a client who was suspicious that her nanny might be neglecting her child. She decided to do a little of her own detective work and place a "nanny-cam" in the house. A nanny-cam is a hidden camera that is set to record what goes on at home without the knowledge of your nanny. This particular client discovered that her nanny was doing her own laundry in the afternoons and ignoring the baby crying in the other room. Understandably upset, she confronted the nanny, who proceeded to lie about it. Consequently, that nanny was fired and a better replacement found.

But the ethical dilemma remains—is it okay to record

someone in your home without his or her knowledge? There's no definitive answer to this question. One would certainly hope that you wouldn't have to resort to such tactics, but as I stated before, I believe your child's best interest has to be your primary concern. Just know that if it turns out that your fears were unfounded, and the nanny finds out about the camera, you could stand the chance of losing a good employee. Bottom line: it's a decision all parents have to make for themselves. If your mother's intuition refuses to pipe down and you think that using a nanny-cam will ease your stress level, then a nanny-cam is an option, albeit a controversial one.

Success Story: Shannon

Shannon is a hairdresser and spa owner who used the plan for her two children.

My husband and I were married in November and found out we were expecting in March, so it was a good surprise, but it was a huge surprise! So, I started setting up the plan even before I had the baby.

I like control, and at first I had to learn how to go with all the changes of having a baby. You know, when you start to lose sleep you really start to feel a little bit nutty, like you don't know if you're coming or going. If things don't go your way you start to feel out of control. But now I feel great.

My husband was a little skeptical about The Baby Sleeps Tonight Plan at first, but then as things kicked in and we saw that it worked, he became its biggest fan. He totally believes in it! He's very adamant about it.

This is a way of life for us now; my husband knows it, our nanny knows it, I know it. Our friends pretty much envy us because they see that it works and now they say, "Oh, we have to do that!"

If you're going to have chaos, I like to have organized chaos. You can pretty much accept that with a two-year-old and a seven-month-old things are going to get a bit crazy at times, but everyone always comments on how happy my children are, and how well-behaved they are.

I think the plan is a marriage-saver! We both need our sleep and we like to have our time together. I mean we were just married and having a good old time when we found out we were pregnant. And with The Baby Sleeps Tonight Plan, we can still have that. Since we know the kids go to bed at eight o'clock, we can just throw some steaks on the grill, go out on the back patio, and have a date night whenever we want to.

I have two sisters who don't use the plan and they're always giving me a hard time, like "Oh, you and your plan," but I really feel like I get the last laugh because you can see that it's working.

The Baby Sleeps Tonight Plan saved me in many ways. It made me enjoy my children from the beginning, not be scared of them, and not be intimidated to try new things.

Also it kept my husband and me from falling into some traps like taking the baby into bed with us. We have the confidence to know that our babies are secure and happy and that's just amazing to us.

This plan has absolutely, 100 percent made us better parents.

Chapter 11

Troubleshooting

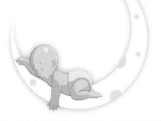

YOUR QUESTIONS ANSWERED

Even though we may often feel alone in our experiences as new parents, in actuality we all share the same emotions and challenges. In my years as a sleep schedule specialist, I've encountered many specific questions from clients that can be of value for you and your family. Here are some of the most commonly asked questions:

My baby is waking up in the middle of the night and I've been trying to evaluate the cause. I have noticed that he hasn't had a poopie diaper in two days. Could this be the problem?

Definitely. If you're a breast-feeding mom I would recommend increasing the fiber in your diet since everything that goes through you goes to your baby. You might also try some gentle exercise techniques with your baby, such as moving his legs in a bicycle motion. If this doesn't fix

202 THE BABY SLEEPS TONIGHT

the problem, I would recommend checking with your pediatrician for advice.

My mother is a strict believer in feeding-on-demand, which was popular when my brother and I were young, and she's totally resistant to The Baby Sleeps Tonight Plan. How can I convince her that this is what we want to do?

First, you have to understand that your mother is operating from the only frame of reference she knows—her own experience. The old equation was: crying baby + feeding = quiet baby. What she doesn't know is that with this plan we're meeting the baby's needs ahead of time with efficient feedings. In any case, you're probably not going to change your mother's philosophy, but you can explain why this plan is important to you and ask that she be supportive of your decision.

I was in the hospital for an extended period of time and wasn't able to use the plan right from the beginning. Can I still get my baby on The Baby Sleeps Tonight Plan?

Absolutely, jump right in! However, sooner is better than later, because you'll avoid having to overcome any established patterns of conditioning (i.e., baby cries, bottle is inserted, baby is quiet). We want to avoid building an expectation in the baby that whenever he cries he gets pacified; we want him to learn to self-soothe.

I'm a single mother and I have no help at all. Can I still use The Baby Sleeps Tonight Plan?

Yes, but you'll NEED to sleep when the baby sleeps. This is very important! Since you'll have to be responsible for doing all the feedings yourself, getting your rest has to be your number-one priority! But don't worry; this grueling pace is only temporary, and by the end of the sixth week you'll be close to "easy street." With The Baby Sleeps Tonight Plan you will reach your goal in the shortest amount of time possible.

My two-year-old is so jealous of the new baby that he's clamoring for my attention all the time and making it hard for me to stick to the plan. What can I do?

It's important to remember that your older child's needs haven't changed just because your life has. Carve out some special "mommy and me" time to help ease the transition into being an older sibling. Reassure the child of your love and explain that he is still important to you. Finally, allow the older child to help out with the new baby. Doing so can foster a sense of pride and accomplishment in the older child and help to lessen the feeling of competition.

It's my birthday and I really love Italian food, but I'm a breast-feeding mom. Can I splurge just this once and still breast-feed without upsetting my baby's digestive system and keep on The Baby Sleeps Tonight Plan?

Happy birthday! Go out and have an awesome time! Life is about living, and every now and then you'll want to go out and celebrate! Let's say you and your husband go to your favorite Italian restaurant and share a bottle of red wine, a Caesar salad, pasta with marinara sauce, and chocolate flambé. That's fine, enjoy every bite, but my advice would be to go home and pump and dump. If you give that milk to your baby, his immature digestive system will feel the effects and consequently disrupt his sleep. Give yourself a treat but give the baby either formula or breast milk that you've pumped ahead of time. Pumping and dumping for just one feeding should do it. You'll be as good as new for the next one!

I'm having trouble waking my baby to feed; what can I do?

This is quite common with younger babies and will get easier as the baby gets older. The idea here is to make the baby less comfortable. Try any of the following techniques to stimulate your baby: change your baby's diaper; take a cool washcloth and touch the forehead or tickle the toes; insert a bottle or nipple in a front-to-back or side-to-side motion; or take your baby's clothes off and go skin to skin.

My baby wakes up crying in her crib before the scheduled feeding time. What do I do?

First, go through your Crying Checklist (see page 70). Then, if all your baby's needs have been met, you have a choice—you can either wait until the scheduled time to go in, or go in and try to soothe your baby in the crib without picking her up. You do not want to pick her up because she will associate crying with being picked up. Once she is soothed and not crying you can pick her up. Take her out and play or dance with her in order to stretch the time to the next feeding.

My baby is already six weeks old and I just found out about the plan. Is it too late to begin?

No, start right in on feeding every three hours, and examine your baby's wake-time. If you're able to keep him up for the full hour, including that thirty-minute wake-time, and you're able to get the baby to sleep from midnight to 6:00 a.m., you're right on track. If it takes a couple of weeks to get into the swing of things, don't worry about it! Just make sure your baby sleeps from midnight until 6:00 a.m. before you move to the next goal. The Baby Sleeps Tonight Plan is designed as a guide to get baby onboard no matter what stage he or she is at. Just stick with it!

My baby is sick with a cold. Can I still stay on the schedule?

When a baby is sick you have to take care of your child first and if it means deviating from the schedule, then you must do that. Try to stay as close to the schedule as possible, however, and then when baby is well, get right back on track. You can expect that it might take two to three days to get back on schedule. This is perfectly normal.

How do I plan my doctor's appointments and still adhere to the plan?

Try to schedule your appointments around your baby's wake-time if possible. Plan to drive when she is sleeping and feed when you get there. That way, she will be awake during your appointment and ready for another nap when you get back in the car.

I'm in the car and my baby is crying in the backseat. How can I get him back to sleep?

Use the magic of the rhythm to help soothe the moment! Turn on rap music or something with a strong beat and you'll see your baby relax or calm down. Remember, babies love a beat because it simulates the sounds that they heard in the womb, so use this fact to your advantage! Your baby will be back to sleep in no time.

My husband has been sweet enough to take over the bedtime feeding so that I can get some extra sleep. The problem is, when my son wakes in the middle of the night, how can I be sure that he's been efficiently fed since I didn't do the feeding?

First, it's wonderful for both you and your child that your husband is taking such an active role in the plan! The fix for this dilemma is easy. Since your husband is bottle-feeding your son, just instruct him to leave the bottle on the nightstand next to you when he's done. That way, if the baby wakes in the night, one quick glance at the bottle will tell you just how much breast milk or formula your son consumed. Again, if your child continues to wake in the night and you're using breast milk for the bedtime feeding, you might try switching to formula to see if that keeps your baby feeling satisfied longer.

Should I continue to allow my child to use a pacifier in order to get to sleep?

My philosophy is to use them just occasionally. If you always use one to calm your baby, then you'll always need it. Use other tools and techniques to soothe your baby, such as rhythmic patting and shushing, rubbing your baby's head, comforting touch, or repetitive words. You can allow your baby to use your knuckle as a substitute for the pacifier for a few moments if needed. The warmth of a mother's touch is so powerful. Even the slightest contact can have an amazing effect on your child.

My child is not sleeping through the night and I think it's because she's having a hard time burping.

If your baby hasn't been burped effectively that most certainly could affect her sleeping. When burping your baby, make sure that you have the baby vertical, high on your breastbone. Then pat her firmly and rhythmically so that you can help work up any gas bubbles that may be causing discomfort. There are several different ways to burp your baby, but I find that holding the baby high on the breastbone creates a hard surface which allows this technique to be the most effective. In time, you'll find just the right technique to ease your baby into a peaceful sleep.

My daughter is right on schedule during the day and feeds every three and a half hours, but at night she's still waking up at 3:00 a.m. What could be the problem?

First, did baby efficiently feed at the bedtime feeding? Refer back to the "How Much Should I Feed My Baby?" section in chapter 3. If you're breast-feeding you should review what you've eaten recently to see if that could be causing gastrointestinal distress in the baby. Another possibility is that you may have inadvertently created an unfavorable pattern by responding to your daughter's crying too quickly. Once you've thoroughly evaluated the possibilities, take the necessary actions to remedy the situation as soon as possible.

My baby is three months old; how much should I be feeding her at this stage?

Every child is different and unique. If you're breast-feeding your child, you should be able to drain both breasts in thirty minutes. If you're feeding with formula, children at this age (three months) typically consume six to eight ounces per feeding. No two children are the same, of course, but as a general rule, little boys seem to drink more than little girls, perhaps because of their size difference.

My friends tell me that adding rice cereal to a bottle with the formula will help my eight-week-old sleep longer. Should I do it?

If you've been using The Baby Sleeps Tonight Plan then no rice cereal should be necessary because your baby will already be sleeping through the night at this stage. Feeding after the evening nap (the bedtime feeding) takes hunger out of the equation. However, if you decide that you'd like to try introducing rice cereal to your baby, I would recommend checking with your pediatrician as to the appropriate time to begin adding solid foods.

My baby is nine weeks old. Should he be taking all his naps in the crib?

At this stage, I would recommend that your baby take at least one nap a day in the crib in order to keep him grounded and familiar in that environment. Let him know that it is his special place. However, if your baby falls asleep in a stroller or bouncy seat, let him finish his nap there. You only have a short window of opportunity within which to move your child, while in the early stages of sleep (the first twenty minutes); otherwise it can disturb the sleep pattern.

How can we go out to dinner as a family without disrupting our baby's schedule?

Plan your reservation time around the baby's feeding. Feed the baby at the restaurant, and then you'll have the baby hanging out with you during his wonderful wake-time. By the time you're ready to leave, your baby will be ready to sleep in the car on the way home.

My husband and I are going out on a date and have a ba-by-sitter. How do I make sure the baby-sitter stays on our schedule? I'm a bit worried that she won't follow my plan.

If she doesn't follow the plan you'll know it right away because the baby will wake earlier than usual. Not to worry though, it will only take a day or so to get back in the groove, if that's the case. Remember, if you fall off the schedule you can always get back on track because you have a guideline. Just start your day again at 7:00 a.m. (I might also suggest finding another baby-sitter.)

How do I travel across time zones and manage to keep my baby on the schedule?

If you're only going across one time zone, stick to the original plan and just get up an hour earlier or later. If it's more than one time zone, and you choose to adapt your baby to the new time, then just know that you'll have to work a bit to get her back on the original schedule once you get home. The longer you're off of the schedule, the longer it takes to get back on it, but as usual, consistency will see you through.

I like the nanny I interviewed but I'm not sure that my son will feel the same way. What should I do?

I'd recommend having your child spend some quality time with the nanny before making a long-term commitment. Perhaps you could audition your candidate beforehand by having them do a trial week or some baby-sitting to make sure it's a good fit.

My son has always been wonderful on the plan, but lately when I'm putting him to bed after day care, he's not even interested in going to sleep! I can't manage to get him to sleep until 10:30 p.m.! Help!

If your little man isn't interested in sleeping at his bedtime, chances are your day care isn't following The Baby Sleeps Tonight Plan. Most likely they're letting him nap longer than his usual naptime. You may want to consider "popping in" at the day care, at the end of naptime, to see if he's still being allowed to sleep. If so, talk to the day-care provider and emphasize your desire to keep him on a specific schedule.

Help!!! My nine-month-old was sleeping great and now is having a hard time going to sleep. What is going on with him?

A nine-month-old is going through lots of changes. He's probably crawling all over the place, possibly teething, and also eating solids. First, I would look at his sugar intake. Try to eliminate sugar (including fruits) after 3:00 p.m. Also, as an energetic young boy he might just need some additional wind-down time before bed. Try doing a family circle, reading your child a story, and then allowing him to listen to some soft music until he falls asleep.

My one-and-a-half-year-old missed going down for her afternoon nap and it is now 4:00 p.m. Do I put her to bed early or give her a nap now?

My recommendation would be to give a short nap (only twenty-five minutes) and then wake her up. This will give her a short amount of rest and will ensure a good night's sleep on time. If she takes longer than twenty-five minutes, know that she will be going down later than her designated bedtime. Another example would be if you let her sleep for one hour at 4:00 p.m., don't try to put her to sleep at her designated bedtime. Delay it by one hour.

My one-and-a-half-year-old wants me to read multiple books to her every night before she'll go to sleep. I'm so tired from working all day that I can only manage to read her one. Can you recommend a solution for me?

Creating balance at home is hard especially after a long day at work. Here's a great solution: read her one book, then put her to bed and put on an audio book for her to listen to until she falls asleep. Audio books are a wonderful option and a great compromise for both of you.

My friend allows her two-year-old to have a sip of soda as a treat. I don't think that's a good idea because I know that sugar can affect sleep. Do you have any alternatives?

As a matter of fact, I do! There are wonderful flavor-infused seltzers out there. No sugar, no calories, no problem! Tell your child that they are having "pop" and they will learn to acquire a taste for something natural. For example, I gave my kids Perrier and called it "lemon pop" and they loved it! It's best if you can avoid rewarding your children with sugary treats. You can do the same thing with "cookies." Give your child cheese crackers and call them "cheese cookies"! Your child will still feel like he's received something special, and will learn to turn to healthier alternatives in the long run.

How do we handle The Baby Sleeps Tonight Plan in regard to special occasions with my two-year-old?

Special occasions should not be missed! Remember it is about overall sleep and overall wake-time. So, if you want your child to stay up later in the evening past his bedtime, give him an "extra" nap in the late afternoon for no more than one hour so he can be fresh for your evening event. Then delay bedtime by one hour.

My husband has been transferred and we're moving to a new home in a month. Is there anything we can do to make the transition easier on our two-year-old so that our sleep schedule won't be disrupted?

Familiarity is the key to happiness and security with a child. They like knowing what to expect. When you set up the new house, try to keep your child's room as similar to the way it was as you can. Use the same bedding and curtains and bring along the same stuffed animals. Most importantly, even though things will understandably be crazy for a while, stick with the schedule. Children crave structure and it will go a long way to helping your child feel comfortable in this new environment.

My child is due for her immunizations. Can I expect to keep her on the schedule during this time?

Getting a shot is an unpleasant fact of life. No matter how you slice it, it hurts! You can expect your child to have some soreness at the injection site and possibly even run a low-grade temperature. If you know ahead of time that your child will be receiving a shot, give her a dose of Tylenol (check with your pediatrician first) before you show up for the appointment, so that it's already working. During the actual injection, distract your child by holding her hands, looking her in the eyes, and talking to her reassuringly. It will be over in no time, and if you can help her to have a positive experience, the next time will be easier. In general, immunizations will not affect the schedule.

My daughter is two and a half and we are preparing for the potty. Our house doesn't have a bathroom in her room. How do I deal with this?

In your situation, you will need to lose your trusted safety gate at this age, and make sure there is a well-lit way to the bathroom in case she needs to go in the middle of the night. Rehearse it with her. This will help, and don't forget to eliminate liquids after 6:00 p.m.!

When my kids watch TV they seem to get wound up and they don't want to go to bed. How should I deal with this?

Television can be a valuable tool, but it should be used in moderation. I recommend no television viewed at least thirty minutes before bed to avoid over-stimulation. However, why not use TV time as a reward? Limiting your child's viewing will make the experience more special. Give your child a couple of suitable options and let him choose what he wants to watch. Many programs geared toward young children are highly educational and can be helpful with tasks such as learning the alphabet and counting. Limiting television use helps to give positive programming more impact. As long as you strive to create balance in your child's life, television can bring an added dimension by exposing him to people and places he wouldn't ordinarily see. There's a time and a place for everything. Just make sure that sleep time does not involve TV time!

On The Baby Sleeps Tonight Plan, how do I handle the switch to Daylight Savings Time and back to Standard Time?

It takes about two to three days to get back on track. For "springing forward" to Daylight Savings Time, the night you will be changing the clocks, try moving bedtime 30 minutes earlier. Wake baby at 7:00 a.m. as usual to feed. For "falling back" to Standard Time, try to put baby to bed 30 minutes later than usual. Note that baby might wake earlier than usual. Try to hold baby off to feed until at least 6:30 a.m., then the next day, try to get closer to 7:00 a.m.

WHAT IF MY BABY...

wakes early from her nap?

If she has been napping for less than forty-five minutes, you may go in and try to soothe her with rhythmic patting, rubbing, and shushing while she's still in the crib to transition her back to sleep. Do not stay in longer than five minutes.

won't go down at the beginning of the nap?

Try to relax your baby before putting him down for the nap. Use soft music, baby massage, and rocking to help transition to nap. See chapter 4, "Preparing Baby for the Nap."

misses a nap?

It's not the end of the world! Don't worry, just make up the time later on during the day with the next nap. Add extra time on to that nap but don't miss the next feeding.

is totally off the schedule?

You have a guide. Get back to the designated feeding and nap schedule and you will be back on schedule within two days.

is taking a long time to breast-feed?

First, make sure you're breast-feeding correctly. Newborns will need to be taught to feed even though they have the natural reflex to suck. Keeping your baby up to feed is key. Resort back to techniques for keeping baby awake in chapter 4.

is crying after a feeding?

Go back to the Crying Checklist, chapter 4.

is chewing on the nipple during bottle- and breast-feeding?

Your baby is probably cutting a tooth. See the section in chapter 8 titled "Prescription for Teething."

refuses a bottle while weaning off exclusive breast-feeding?

Work on giving a bottle at the first feeding of the day when the baby is very hungry. If you are weaning off breast-feeding, don't cut it out "cold-turkey"; simply ease off of it and your baby and breasts will thank you.

seems hungry after an efficient thirty-minute breast-feeding and both breasts have been drained?

If your baby is four months old or older, try supplementing with two ounces of formula/breast milk from a bottle after the feeding. Chances are breast milk production may be declining if your baby drinks the two ounces. If your baby is younger than four months old, see chapter 3 for breast-feeding advice.

can't stop passing gas?

Check chapter 3 for the section "Fighting Fussiness and Gas."

starts crying in the car while driving?

Put on the radio and tune in to a station that plays rap music or something with a strong beat. This will calm the baby down.

falls asleep in the car for thirty minutes before scheduled naptime?

Delay next naptime by thirty minutes.

Conclusion

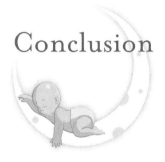

Sleep is one of our body's most important functions. Regular, high-quality sleep has wonderful effects on your overall health and sense of well-being. Studies have shown that rested individuals show improved performance on tasks like problem-solving, memory retention, and handling stress. By implementing The Baby Sleeps Tonight Plan in your life, you have eliminated sleep deprivation, one of the biggest challenges standing in the way of your family's predictable happiness. The plan has put control back into your hands, and the positive effects of structure on a child's behavior are immeasurable. Having a familiar routine builds confidence, decreases anxiety and fear, and encourages cooperation, as well as compliance. When a child can anticipate future events, it increases his sense of control and independence. The long-term rewards of The Baby Sleeps Tonight Plan are far-reaching:

- It promotes a feeling of security in your child. This is especially true for younger children who need routines in order to feel secure in their environment.
- You can better plan your day. By having a moment-by-moment outline of your daily schedule, you'll know exactly what times you're available and won't be running late because your child has suddenly fallen asleep just before you set off on an errand.
- You have more quality time for yourself and your partner. All new parents will inevitably go through an adjustment period while getting used to their new roles. For this reason, it's crucial for you and your partner to carve out some couple-time to nurture your changing relationship. The plan protects and preserves the foundation of your family's happiness—your intimate relationship—by allowing you to tangibly make time for one of the most important people in your life.
- You strengthen family relationships. With scheduled mealtimes and bedtime rituals, parents and children are encouraged to spend quality time together on a regular basis, and not just when an opportunity happens to present itself.
- It promotes wellness. Not only does maintaining a regular, healthy sleep pattern help you to be happier, but it also helps you to be healthier. Sleep deprivation can weaken your immune system so that your body has a harder time fighting off viruses and infections. By making sure that

everyone in your family is well rested, you're also taking steps to ensure each member's good health.

- You're creating a positive pattern that will last a lifetime. Your child doesn't need to be a toddler in order to appreciate a routine. Children of all ages benefit from having a schedule. With the plan, you've given your child a love of order and organization. Setting goals and defining priorities will come more naturally to children who have been raised on a schedule. The independence, self-control, and dependability they've learned are lessons that will stay with them for the rest of their lives.

As you can see, the benefits of The Baby Sleeps Tonight Plan are many. Although the rewards start with a great night's sleep, the end result is predictable happiness for you and your family. Parenthood doesn't have to be so challenging! Congratulations for taking the first steps toward empowering yourself and your children, and welcome to *The Baby Sleeps Tonight* family. Here's wishing you and your entire family a happy, prosperous, and well-rested future!

The Baby Sleeps Tonight
Plan At-a-Glance

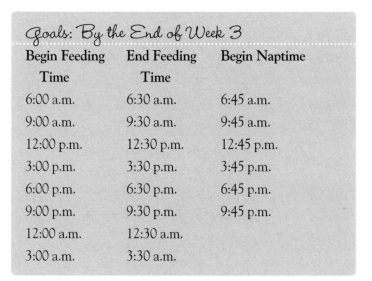

Goals: By the End of Week 3

Begin Feeding Time	End Feeding Time	Begin Naptime
6:00 a.m.	6:30 a.m.	6:45 a.m.
9:00 a.m.	9:30 a.m.	9:45 a.m.
12:00 p.m.	12:30 p.m.	12:45 p.m.
3:00 p.m.	3:30 p.m.	3:45 p.m.
6:00 p.m.	6:30 p.m.	6:45 p.m.
9:00 p.m.	9:30 p.m.	9:45 p.m.
12:00 a.m.	12:30 a.m.	
3:00 a.m.	3:30 a.m.	

Goals: By the End of Week 6

Begin Feeding Time	End Feeding Time	Begin Naptime
6:00 a.m.	6:30 a.m.	7:00 a.m.
9:00 a.m.	9:30 a.m.	10:00 a.m.
12:00 p.m.	12:30 p.m.	1:00 p.m.
3:00 p.m.	3:30 p.m.	4:00 p.m.
6:00 p.m.	6:30 p.m.	7:00 p.m.
9:00 p.m.	9:30 p.m.	10:00 p.m.
12:00 a.m.	12:30 a.m.	

Goals: Weeks 7 and 8

STAGE 1

Begin Feeding Time	End Feeding Time	Begin Naptime
6:00 a.m.	6:30 a.m.	7:10 a.m.
9:30 a.m.	10:00 a.m.	10:40 a.m.
1:00 p.m.	1:30 p.m.	2:10 p.m.
4:30 p.m.	5:00 p.m.	5:40 p.m.
8:00 p.m.	8:30 p.m.	9:10 p.m.
11:30 p.m.	12:00 a.m.	

STAGE 2

Begin Feeding Time	End Feeding Time	Begin Naptime
6:30 a.m.	7:00 a.m.	7:50 a.m.
10:00 a.m.	10:30 a.m.	11:20 a.m.
1:30 p.m.	2:00 p.m.	2:50 p.m.
5:00 p.m.	5:30 p.m.	6:20 p.m.
8:30 p.m.	9:00 p.m.	10:00 p.m.–11:00 p.m. 1-Hour Nap
11:30 p.m.	12:00 a.m.	

STAGE 3

Begin Feeding Time	End Feeding Time	Begin Naptime
6:30 a.m.	7:00 a.m.	8:00 a.m.
10:00 a.m.	10:30 a.m.	11:30 a.m.
1:30 p.m.	2:00 p.m.	3:00 p.m.
5:00 p.m.	5:30 p.m.	6:30 p.m.
8:30 p.m.	9:00 p.m.	9:30 p.m.–10:30 p.m. 1-Hour Nap
11:00 p.m.	11:30 p.m.	

Goals: Weeks 9 Onward

STAGE 1

Begin Feeding Time	Designated Naptime
7:00 a.m.	8:45 a.m.
11:00 a.m.	12:45 p.m.
3:00 p.m.	**5:15 p.m.–6:15 p.m.**
7:00 p.m.	**8:30 p.m.–9:30 p.m.**
11:00 p.m.	

STAGE 2

Begin Feeding Time	Designated Naptime
7:00 a.m.	8:45 a.m.
11:00 a.m.	12:45 p.m.
3:00 p.m.	**5:15 p.m.–6:15 p.m.**
7:00 p.m.	**8:30 p.m.–9:30 p.m.**
10:30 p.m.	

STAGE 3

Begin Feeding Time	Designated Naptime
7:00 a.m.	8:45 a.m.
11:00 a.m.	12:45 p.m.
3:00 p.m.	**5:15 p.m.–6:15 p.m.**
6:45 p.m.	
10:15 p.m.	

Stage 4

Begin Feeding Time	Designated Naptime
7:00 a.m.	8:45 a.m.
11:00 a.m.	12:45 p.m.
3:00 p.m.	**5:15 p.m.–6:15 p.m.**
6:30 p.m.	
10:00 p.m.	

Stage 5

Begin Feeding Time	Designated Naptime
7:00 a.m.	8:45 a.m.
11:00 a.m.	12:45 p.m.
3:00 p.m.	**5:00 p.m.–6:00 p.m.**
6:15 p.m.	
9:45 p.m.	

Stage 6

Begin Feeding Time	Designated Naptime
7:00 a.m.	8:45 a.m.
11:00 a.m.	12:45 p.m.
3:00 p.m.	**4:45 p.m.–5:45 p.m.**
6:00 p.m.	
9:30 p.m.	

Note: Based on 7:00 a.m. wake up.

Note: Bold indicates times that are changing in weeks 9 onward.

ULTIMATE SCHEDULE

Begin Feeding Time	Designated Naptime
7:00 a.m.	8:45 a.m.
11:00 a.m.	12:45 p.m.
3:00 p.m.	**4:45 p.m.–5:45 p.m.**
6:00 p.m.	
9:00 p.m. (or earlier)	

Note: Based on 7:00 a.m. wake up.

Note: Bold indicates times that are changing in weeks 9 onward.

Appendix B

Sources

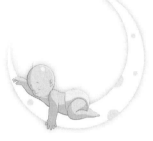

Introduction

Sleep: Talkaboutsleep.com. An Intro to Sleep: What is Sleep? http://www.talkaboutsleep.com/sleep-disorders/archives/intro.htm.

Chapter 1

Cord Blood Registry: Cord Blood Registry. http://www.cordblood.com/index.asp.

Dogs and babies: The Humane Society of the United States. Introducing Your Pet and New Baby. http://www.hsus.org/pets/pet_care/introducing_your_pet_and_new_baby.html.

Cats and babies: McCarthy, Claudine. Cat Meets Baby. http://www.sthuberts.org/petpouri/articles/catmeetsbaby.asp.

Average adult sleep needs: National Sleep Foundation. How Much Sleep Do We Really Need? http://www.sleepfoundation.org/how-much-sleep-do-we-really-need.

Chapter 2

Baby blues: The Baby Center. The Baby Blues. http://www
.babycenter.com/0_the-baby-blues_11704.bc.

Postpartum depression: Epperson, C. Neill, MD. Postpartum
Major Depression: Detection and Treatment. http://www
.aafp.org/afp/990415ap/2247.html.

Depression help resources: U.S. Department of Health and
Human Services. Depression During and After Pregnancy:
A Resource for Women, Their Families, and Friends.
http://mchb.hrsa.gov/pregnancyandbeyond/depression/
help.htm.

Chapter 3

How much formula?: Babycenter.com . How to tell how
much formula your baby needs. http://www.babycenter.
com/0_how-to-tell-how-much-formula-your-baby-
needs_9136.bc.

Colostrum: La Leche League International. What is colostrum? How does it benefit my baby? http://www.llli.org/
FAQ/colostrum.html.

Mother's Milk Tea: Kellymom Breast-feeding and Parenting.
Herbal Remedies for Increasing Milk Supply. http://www
.kellymom.com/herbal/milksupply/herbal-rem_j.html.

LIPIL Formulas: California WIC Branch. Infant Formula
Supplemented with Fatty Acids. http://www.calwic.org/
docs/federal/lipil.pdf.

Playtex Drop-Ins: Viewpoints. Playtex Drop-Ins Original Nurser Baby Bottle Reviews. http://www.viewpoints.com/Playtex-Drop-Ins-Original-Nurser-Baby-Bottle-reviews.

Playtex VentAire bottles: Playtex Baby. VentAire Advanced Bottle System. http://www.playtexbaby.com/Products/Bottles/VentAire.aspx.

BPA-free bottles: Heather Corley. BPA-Free Baby Bottles. http://babyproducts.about.com/od/feedingdrinks/tp/BPA_free_baby_bottles.html.

Colic: MedicineNet.com. Colic. http://www.medicinenet.com/colic/article.htm.

Acid Reflux: Cincinnati Children's Hospital. Gastroesophageal Reflux in Infants. http://www.cincinnatichildrens.org/health/info/newborn/diagnose/ger-infants.htm.

Chapter 4

Crying it out: Ferber, Richard. 2006. *Solve Your Child's Sleep Problems*. New York: Fireside.

Chapter 8

Tongue-thrust reflex: Babycareadvice.com. What are reflexes? http://www.babycareadvice.com/babycare/general_help/article.php?id=41.

Teething: Netdoctor.com. Children's Teeth and Teething. http://www.netdoctor.co.uk/health_advice/facts/teething.htm.

Teething and diarrhea: Babyslumber.com. Teething and Diarrhea: How to help your Baby. http://www.babyslumber.com/articles/baby/teething-and-diarrhea-how-to-help-your-baby.

Benzocaine: Drugs.com. Anesthetics (Dental). http://www.drugs.com/cons/benzocaine-dental.html.

Night terrors: kidshealth.org. What Are Night Terrors? http://kidshealth.org/parent/medical/sleep/terrors.html#.

Potty-training: Mayoclinic.com. Potty training: How to get the job done. http://www.mayoclinic.com/health/potty-training/CC00060.

Potty-training: Iannelli, Vincent, MD. Potty Training. http://www.keepkidshealthy.com/parenting_tips/potty_training/index.html.

Chapter 9

Star charts: KidsBehaviour.co.uk. Using Sticker/Star Charts. http://www.kidsbehaviour.co.uk/UsingStickerStarCharts.html.

Chapter 10

Nannies: International Nanny Association. Frequently Asked Questions: A Nanny for Your Family. http://www.nanny.org/nannyforfamily.php.

Day care: American Academy of Family Physicians. Day Care: Choosing a Good Center. http://familydoctor.org/online/famdocen/home/children/parents/infants/030.html.

Home Day Care: Babycenter.com. Home Day Care: Licensing. http://www.babycenter.com/0_home-daycare-licensing_6038.bc.

Chapter 11

Television: Child Development Institute. Television and Children. http://www.childdevelopmentinfo.com/health_safety/television.shtml.

About the Author

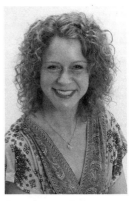

Shari Mezrah is a sleep schedule specialist who has achieved an astonishing 100 percent client success rate with those who have followed her innovative system. She developed her program in 1999 and utilized the plan with her own two children, gaining her the credentials MOM (master's of motherhood). After extensive research, she developed a practical, progressive, and customizable approach. She has assisted hundreds of families and has brought peace and happiness to them all. While her practice BabyTIME is located in Tampa, Florida, she consults with families all over the world through her website www.sharimezrah.com. Her clients include single parents as well as families with multiples.

Shari holds a BA in speech communication from California State University and was the recipient of the prestigious Phi Rho Pi National Speech Honor Society Scholarship. She is a three-time National Forensic Association gold medalist. In 1998 she founded Speakwrite Consulting, a service that provided public speaking coaching to executives. With numerous television appearances to her credit, she is much sought for her baby sleep schedule advice.

Shari is active in many children's organizations. She has served on the board of directors for the Glazer Children's Museum and has been a featured speaker at parent organizations.

She currently resides in Tampa, Florida, with her husband Todd and their children Maxwell and Samantha. The whole Mezrah family is still sleeping through the night!

Notes

Notes